## ACKNOWLEDGEMENTS

To Mother Earth, the eternal source of nourishment and healing.

To my Guru, Bhagawan Sri Sathya Sai Baba, whose divine presence illumines my path.

To Sadguru Sri Madhusudan Sai, with deep love and gratitude, for his constant encouragement, his call to serve others, and his vision that inspires me to honor nature's wisdom in the journey of healing.

To my father, whose unwavering guidance strengthens me.

To my loving and kind family, for always encouraging me, for embracing the natural ways of nourishment, and for patiently being pulled into countless botanical and herbal gardens along the way.

And above all, to the innate intelligence of the Universe, for gifting humanity with plants, herbs, and superfoods—sacred companions in our well-being.

# FOREWORD

Health and healing have always been the natural gifts of Mother Earth. True well-being does not depend on complicated diets or rare ingredients, but on the simple, nourishing foods already within our reach.

In today's world, it is not the lack of resources that distances us from health, but the lack of awareness. Surrounded by processed and addictive foods, we often forget the quiet power of everyday herbs, plants, and natural superfoods.

By bringing these back into our meals with awareness and gratitude, we can meet our body's needs and restore balance and vitality.

Sacred Nourishment is my offering of remembrance—that healing lies not in complexity, but in simplicity, reverence, and a return to Mother Earth's timeless gifts.

# CONTENTS

## THE PROMISE OF THIS BOOK

# "When food is sacred, the body becomes a temple."

This book serves as your comprehensive guide to harnessing the power of eleven renowned plants and foods already integral to Indian culinary traditions. Within its pages, you will delve into the profound spiritual essence of these ingredients, transcending mere scientific data. Moreover, you will gain practical insights into their practical applications, encompassing teas, meals, oils, chutneys, and rituals. Empowered with this knowledge, you will feel confident in nourishing yourself and your family without incurring additional expenses. Furthermore, you will embark on a transformative journey of reconnecting with food as a source of energy, emotion, and wisdom.

It is not necessary for an external authority to dictate what is beneficial for your well-being. Instead, you possess the invaluable gift of remembrance—of the wisdom and knowledge passed down through generations by your ancestors.

# THE POWER OF SUPERFOODS

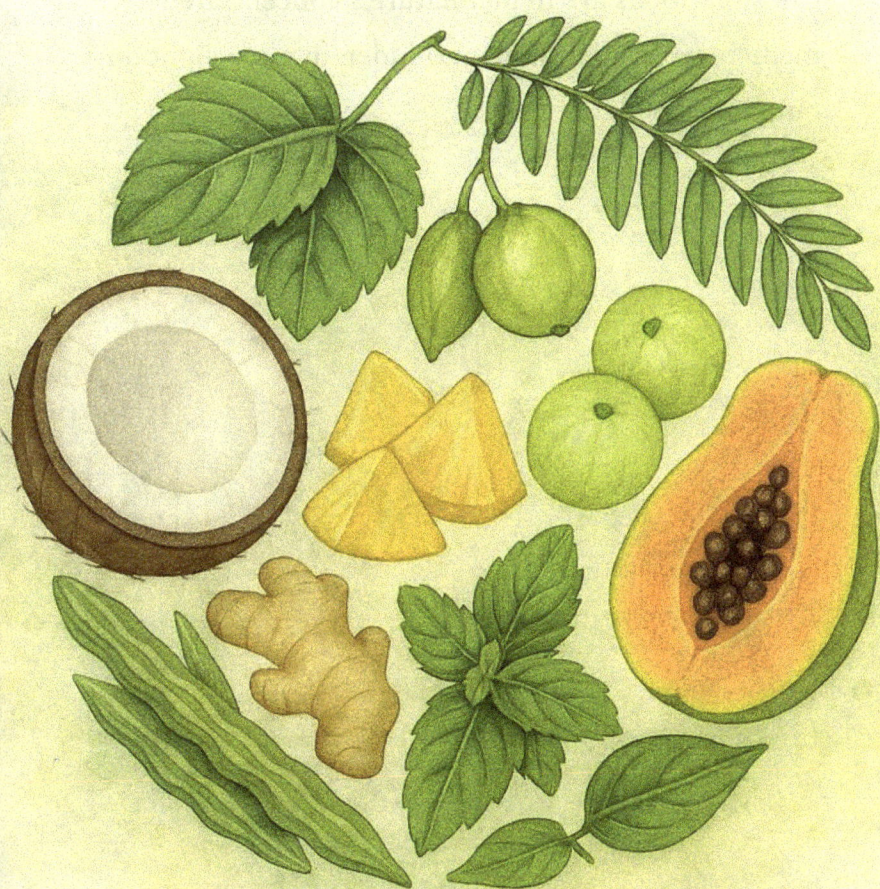

The word "superfood" is popular today, but behind the trend lies a deeper truth — it is where ancient wisdom and modern nutrition science meet. For centuries, traditional systems like Ayurveda have spoken of Rasayana foods — those that rejuvenate the body, calm the mind, and nourish the spirit. In modern science, nutritionists celebrate foods that are nutrient-dense, healing, and preventive. When we put these together, we discover that what we now call superfoods are in fact nature's concentrated medicine and nourishment, hidden in plain sight on our plates.

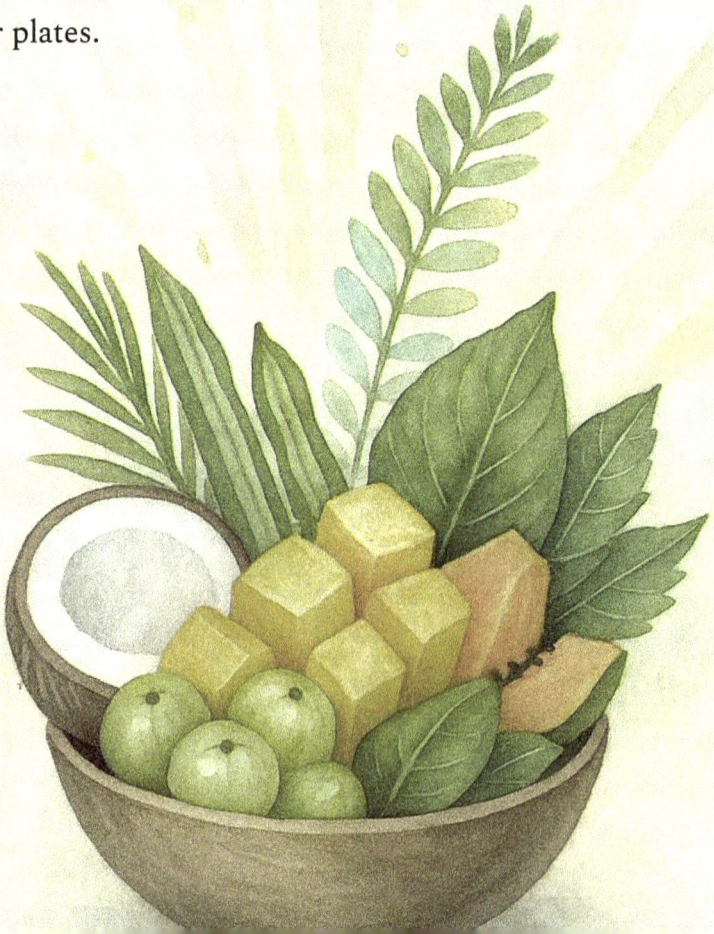

## WHAT MAKES A SUPERFOOD?

A superfood is not a strict scientific label, but rather a recognition of foods that:

- Nourish deeply → rich in vitamins, minerals, antioxidants, or phytonutrients.
- Heal naturally → traditionally used to restore balance, vitality, and immunity.
- Offer more with less → low in calories but high in health-giving compounds.

## EXAMPLES OF SUPERFOODS

### Plant-Based Superfoods

- Amla (Indian Gooseberry) → a powerhouse of Vitamin C, revered for its antioxidant strength.
- Moringa (Drumstick Leaves) → filled with protein, calcium, and iron, known as a "miracle tree."
- Turmeric → with curcumin to reduce inflammation and protect the liver.
- Spinach & Kale → dense in chlorophyll, iron, and folate.

- Blueberries → rich in anthocyanins, guardians of heart and brain health.
- Chia & Flax Seeds → abundant in omega-3 fatty acids and fiber.
- Spirulina → a protein-rich algae with energizing compounds.

## Functional Foods

- Coconut → hydration and healthy fats in one.
- Garlic → protective for the heart, potent against microbes.
- Ginger → a fire for digestion and an antidote to nausea.
- Cinnamon → balancing blood sugar and awakening metabolism.

## Animal-Based Foods (in Some Traditions)

- Yogurt → probiotics for gut harmony.
- Ghee → nourishment for brain and tissues.
- Honey → antimicrobial sweetness from the hive.
- Fatty Fish → abundant in omega-3s for heart and mind.

## WHY SUPERFOODS MATTER

Superfoods protect and restore us in four powerful ways:

1. Shield cells from damage with antioxidants.
2. Balance metabolism — stabilizing blood sugar, hormones, and digestion.
3. Strengthen immunity through vitamins, minerals, and bioactive compounds.
4. Prevent chronic disease such as diabetes, heart disease, and neurodegeneration.

They are not just foods. They are keys to resilience, prevention, and vitality.

## THE ANIMAL PARADOX

Modern veterinary science gives us an interesting mirror. Animals in farms are provided with super-nutrient diets designed to keep them perfectly healthy:

- Prevention over cure → since they cannot communicate illness, their diet is designed to prevent it.

- Efficiency & growth → faster growth, better reproduction, stronger immunity.
- Specialized nutrition → every species gets exactly what it needs — calcium for hens, omega-3 for fish, minerals for cows.
- Human safety → healthier animals mean safer milk, eggs, and meat.

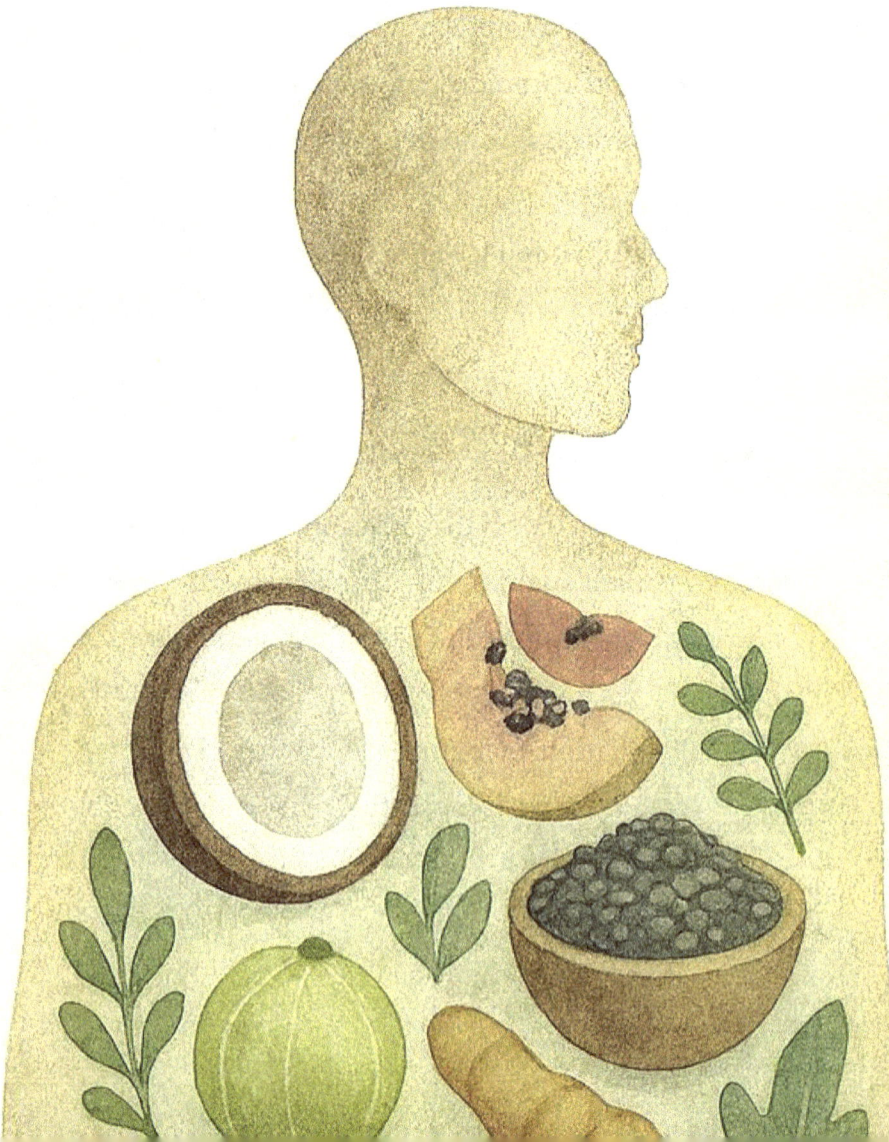

## THE HUMAN IRONY

Humans, on the other hand, often eat the opposite —
processed, nutrient-poor, imbalanced meals. We wait
for sickness before we think of food as medicine.

The irony is striking: while animals are fed
"superfood-level" meals every day to
prevent illness, humans settle for foods that invite
illness in the first place.


## A NEW VISION

What if we flipped this?

What if humans, too, lived on preventive, nutrient-
rich diets that made sickness rare and vitality
natural?

This book is an invitation to reclaim that wisdom —
to feed ourselves as carefully as we feed the creatures
in our care. To embrace superfood diets for
prevention, longevity, and balance.

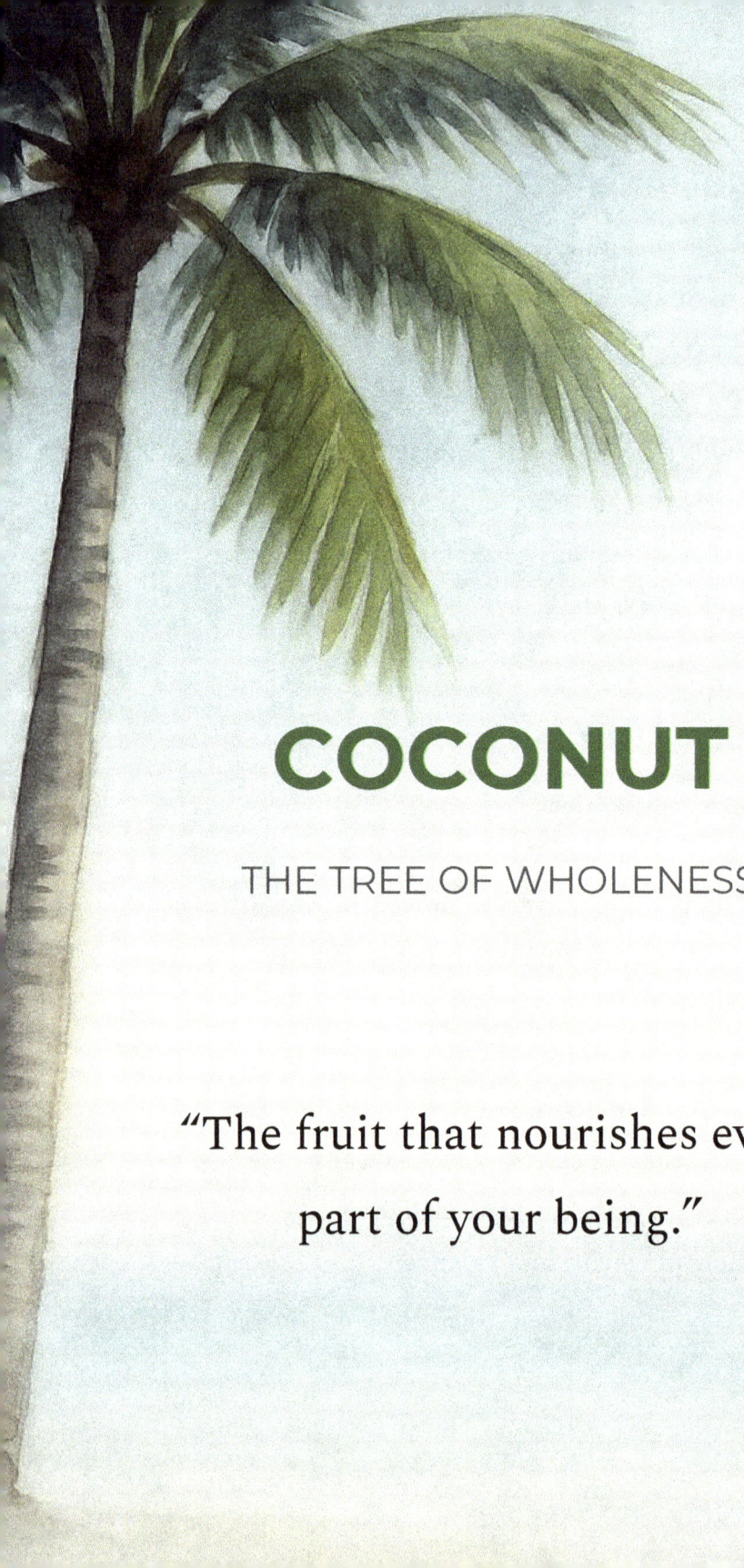

# COCONUT

## THE TREE OF WHOLENESS

"The fruit that nourishes every
part of your being."

## METAPHYSICAL STORY: THE COSMIC TREE OF LIFE

Long ago, when the Earth was still young and the skies were close to the soil, the gods sought a symbol that could carry the essence of abundance, protection, and surrender. They whispered to Mother Earth to birth a tree that would give everything without asking for anything in return. And so, the Coconut Tree was born—its roots deep in the Earth, its head brushing the heavens.

In many ancient traditions, the coconut is seen as the divine offering—used in temples, weddings, and rituals. It is cracked open in front of deities, symbolizing the breaking of ego to reveal the pure self inside.

*The hard outer shell is your worldly armor.*
*The white nourishing flesh is your potential.*
*The sweet water inside is your untouched truth.*

## THE COCONUT TEACHES:

- Be firm on the outside
- Stay soft and nourishing within
- Hold sacred space for inner clarity and sweetness

It is the tree of life in many coastal and tropical traditions, and in Ayurveda, it is considered "Shree Phala"—the fruit of auspiciousness.

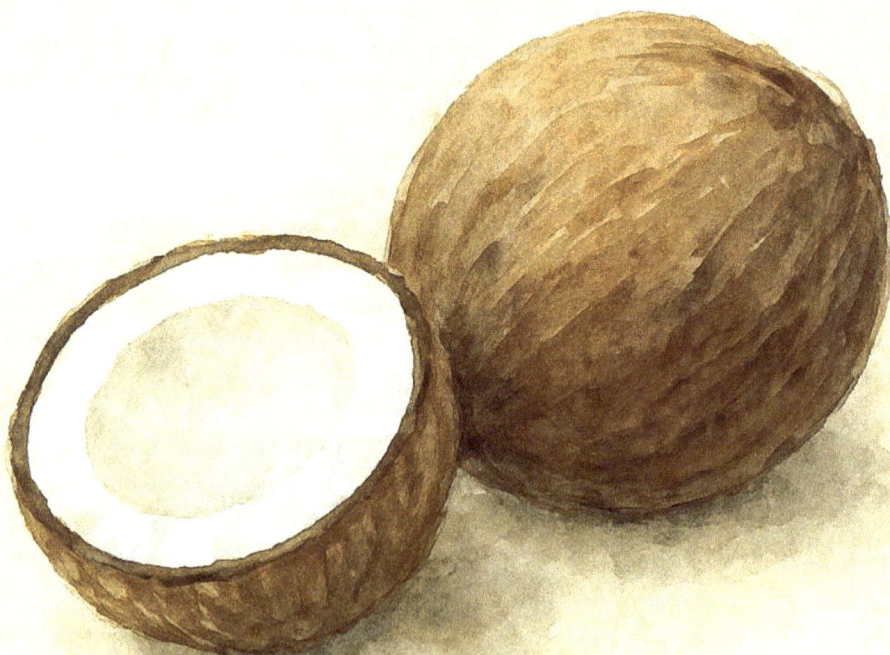

# NUTRITIONAL WHOLENESS OF COCONUT

| Part of Coconut | Nutritional Benefit | Traditional Use |
|---|---|---|
| Coconut Water | Hydrating, rich in potassium & electrolytes | Summer drink, fasting support |
| Tender Coconut Flesh | Easy-to-digest fats, supports gut healing | Weaning food, post-illness nourishment |
| Mature Flesh | Healthy fats (MCTs), fiber, immune boost | Curries, chutneys, sweets |
| Coconut Oil | Antifungal, brain-boosting, hormone-balancing | Hair, skin, cooking, oil pulling |
| Coconut Milk | Calcium, iron, cooling effect | Soups, vegan milk substitute |

Coconut is not just one food—it is many foods in one:

It supports brain health, balances hormones, strengthens the gut, and is excellent for Vata and Pitta doshas.

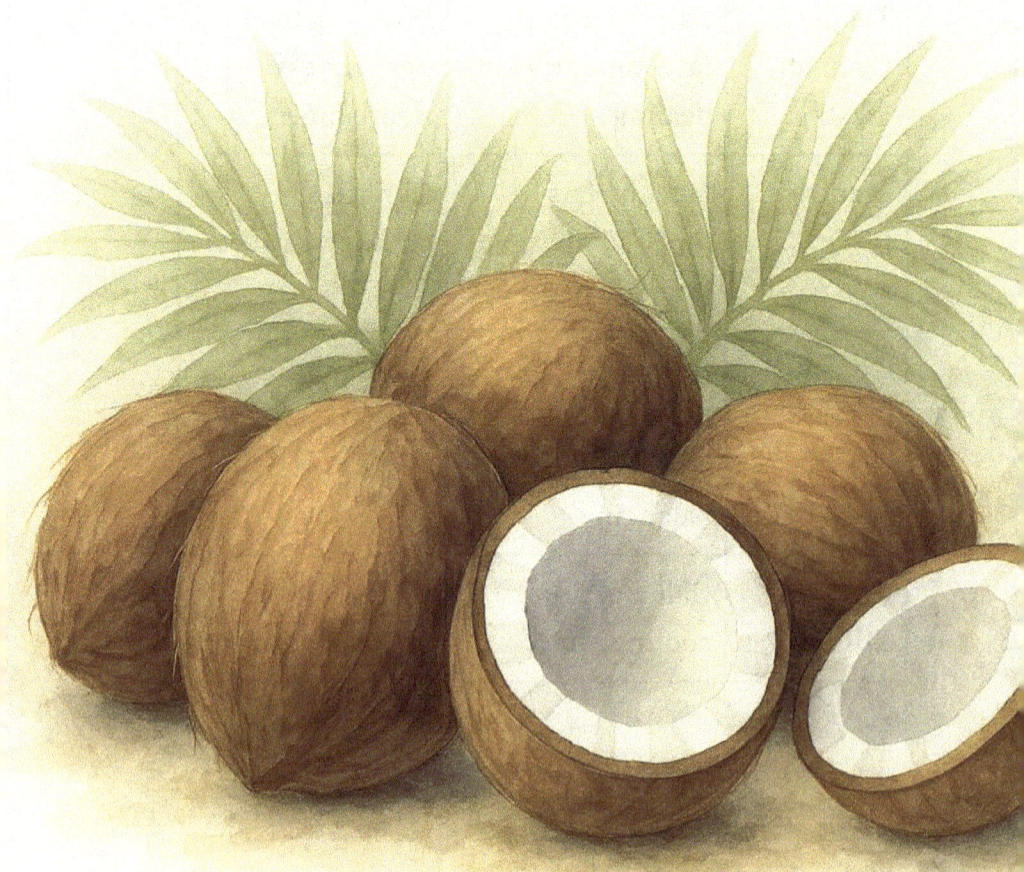

# DAILY RITUALS AND RECIPES WITH COCONUT

Here are some simple, affordable ways to use coconut for nourishment and healing:

## 1. Coconut Chutney

Pair with breakfast idli or dosas.

Blend: grated coconut + green chilies + roasted chana dal + salt + little ginger + water + temper with mustard seeds & curry leaves.

## 2. Oil Pulling (Morning Ritual)

Swish 1 tsp virgin coconut oil in your mouth for 5-10 mins. Spit.

Detoxifies mouth, strengthens gums, clears skin.

## 3. Coconut Milk Khichdi (Cooling)

Cook moong dal and rice with turmeric. Add coconut milk in the end.

Balancing for Pitta, very soothing and nourishing.

### 4. Postpartum Tonic

Roast grated coconut, add jaggery and ghee, make laddoos.

Strengthens bones and uterus after delivery.

## SPIRITUAL PRACTICES

- Place a whole coconut on your home altar.
- Offer it during times of transition, prayer, or new beginnings.
- Break it with intention: "May my ego break, and my true nature flow."

## IN SUMMARY: WHY COCONUT?

☑ Full-spectrum nourishment

☑ Available year-round

☑ Affordable in all Indian regions

☑ Works for body, skin, hormones, gut, and energy

☑ A food of ritual, reverence, and restoration

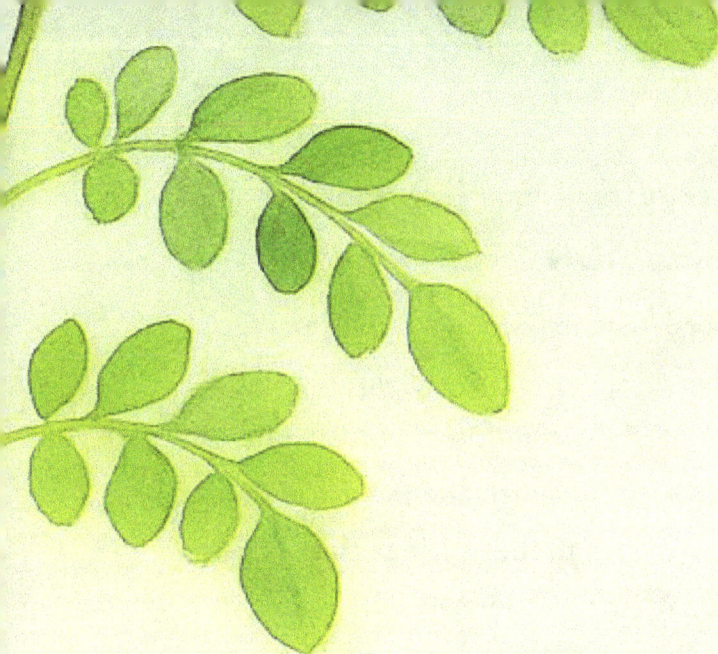

# MORINGA

## THE MIRACLE LEAF OF LIGHT

"A tree that grows in hardship
and nourishes with
abundance."

## METAPHYSICAL STORY: THE RESURRECTION TREE

In Vedic legend, when drought struck and the rivers ran dry, the sages prayed for a plant that could survive the harshest conditions and still offer life. From the dust of the Earth and the fire of the sun, the gods gave birth to the Moringa tree—a being that would not just live, but thrive in scarcity.

The moringa leaf is seen as a symbol of divine grace—small, unassuming, yet bursting with power. It grows fast, needs little, and gives more than it takes. In rural India, it is often planted at the edge of every home, like a quiet guardian.

## MORINGA TEACHES US:

- You can flourish even in adversity
- True strength is quiet, generous, and green
- Nourishment is not about quantity, but depth

# NUTRITIONAL WHOLENESS OF MORINGA

Moringa is considered a complete plant-based multivitamin. Its leaves, pods, flowers, and seeds are all usable.

| Part Used | Nutritional Benefits | Common Use |
|---|---|---|
| Leaves | Protein, iron, calcium, Vitamin A, C, E | Stir-fries, powders, soups |
| Pods (Drumsticks) | Rich in fiber, minerals | Sambhar, curries |
| Seeds | Antioxidants, liver support | Powdered in capsules or oils |
| Flowers | Hormonal balance, energy tonic | Added to curries or teas |

# DAILY RECIPES & RITUALS WITH MORINGA

### 1. Moringa Leaf Stir-Fry (South Indian Style)

Lightly sauté fresh moringa leaves in ghee with mustard seeds, garlic, and grated coconut.
Excellent for fatigue, especially in women and elders.

### 2. Drumstick Sambhar

Add fresh drumsticks to toor dal sambhar with tamarind, turmeric, and curry leaves.
Builds strength and improves digestion.

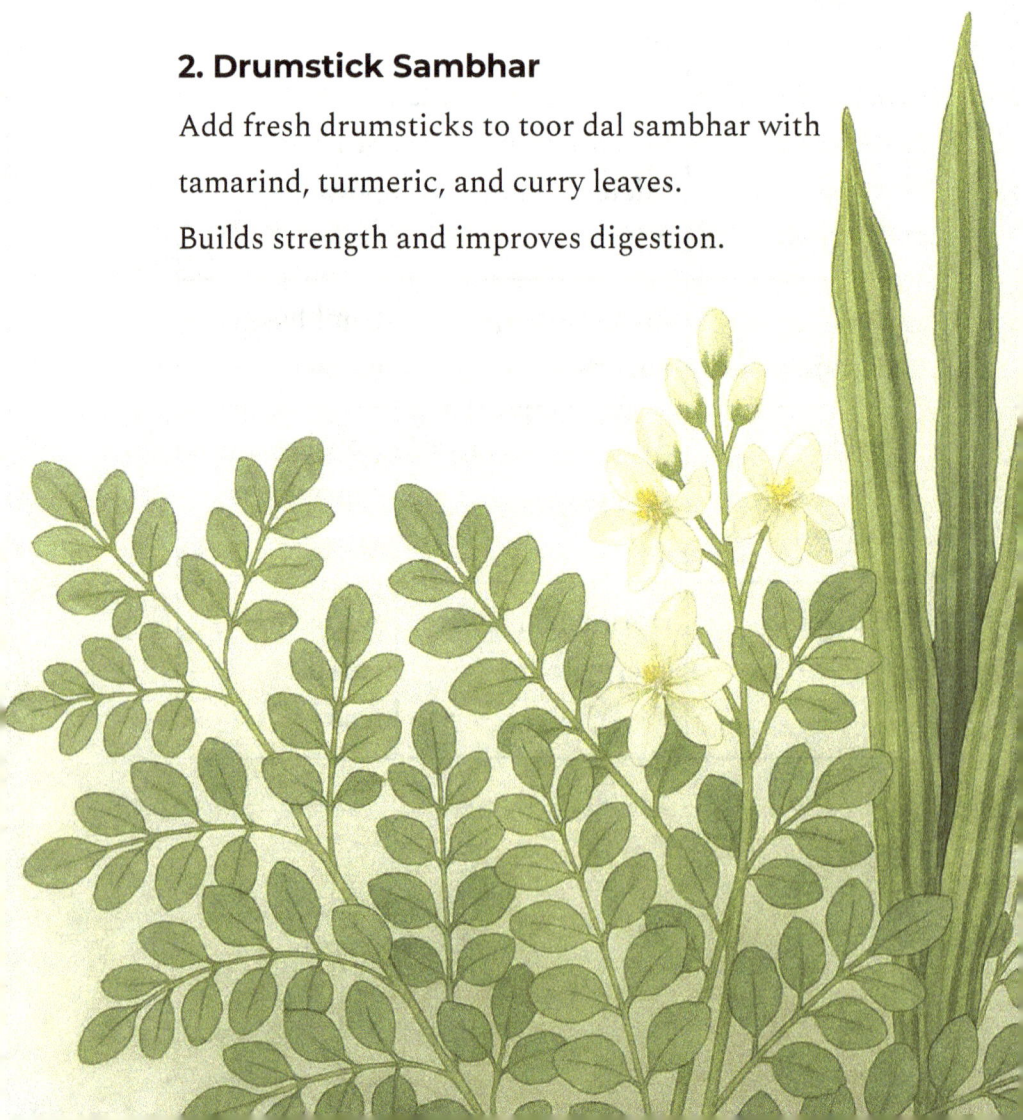

### 3. Moringa Smoothie (Modern twist)

Blend moringa powder with banana, dates, coconut milk, and cardamom.

A complete breakfast—cooling, iron-rich, and energizing.

### 4. Moringa Tea (Detox & Hormone Support)

Steep dried moringa leaves in hot water with ginger and tulsi. Add lemon and jaggery if desired.

Supports liver, reduces inflammation.

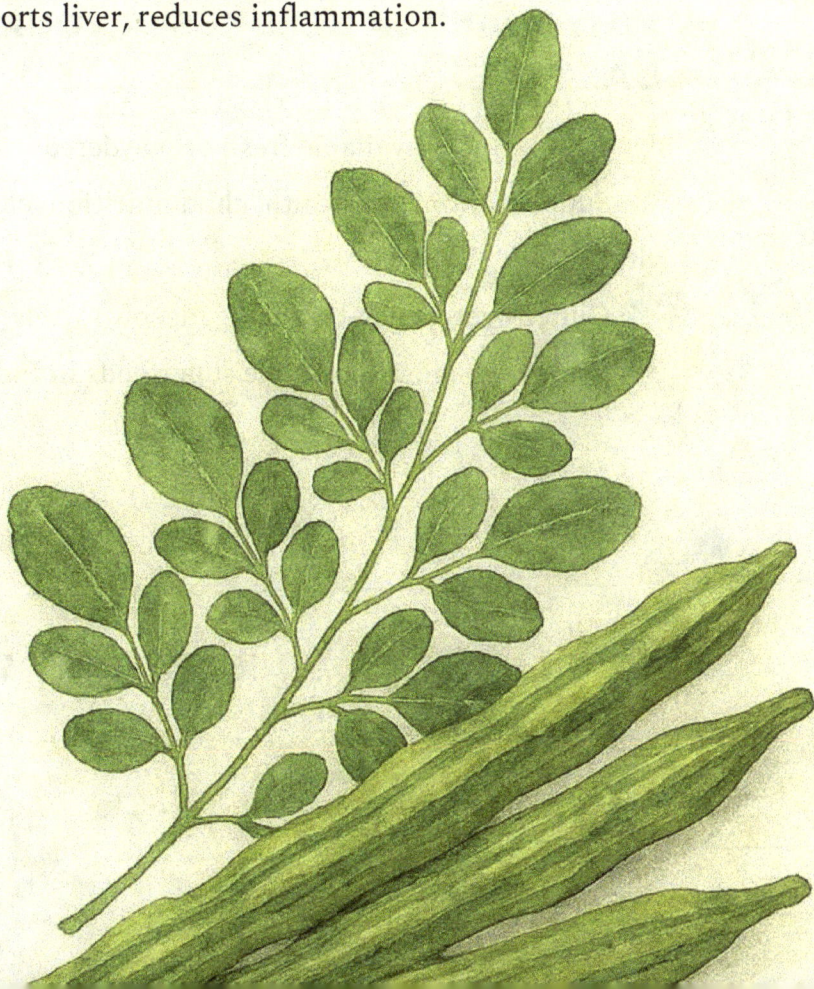

## SPIRITUAL PRACTICES

- Plant a moringa sapling as a ritual of hope, especially after loss or during a new beginning.
- Offer its first leaves to your home altar or deities with the intention: "May my nourishment be rooted in simplicity and service."

## WHY MORINGA BELONGS IN YOUR DAILY DIET

- ✅ Grows easily, available fresh or powdered
- ✅ Supports women's health, child nutrition, elder vitality
- ✅ Gluten-free, sugar-balancing, deeply sattvic
- ✅ One of the most accessible superfoods in India

# JACKFRUIT

## THE GOLDEN FLESH OF VITALITY

"Hidden within a rough armor is the strength and sweetness of life."

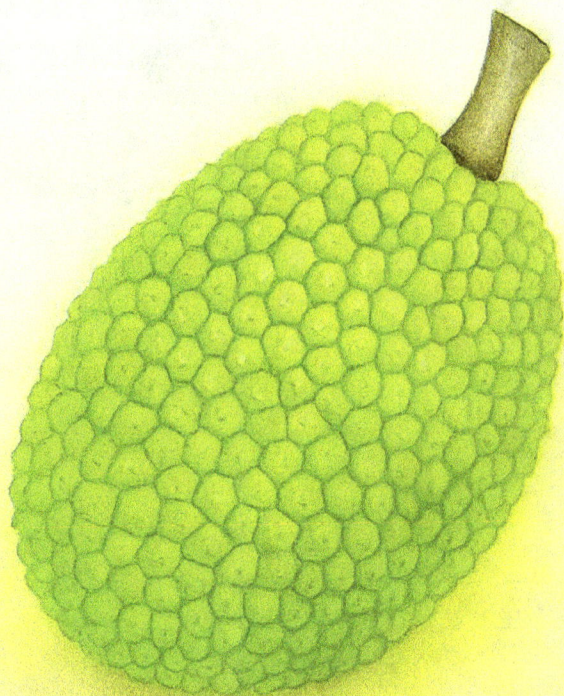

## METAPHYSICAL STORY: THE WARRIOR FRUIT

In ancient lore, the jackfruit was gifted to the forest-dwelling rishis by Mother Earth herself. She shaped it with a tough, spiked shell to protect the soft, golden jewels inside—a lesson in resilience. To taste the sweetness, one had to work through the layers, much like the soul's journey through human trials.

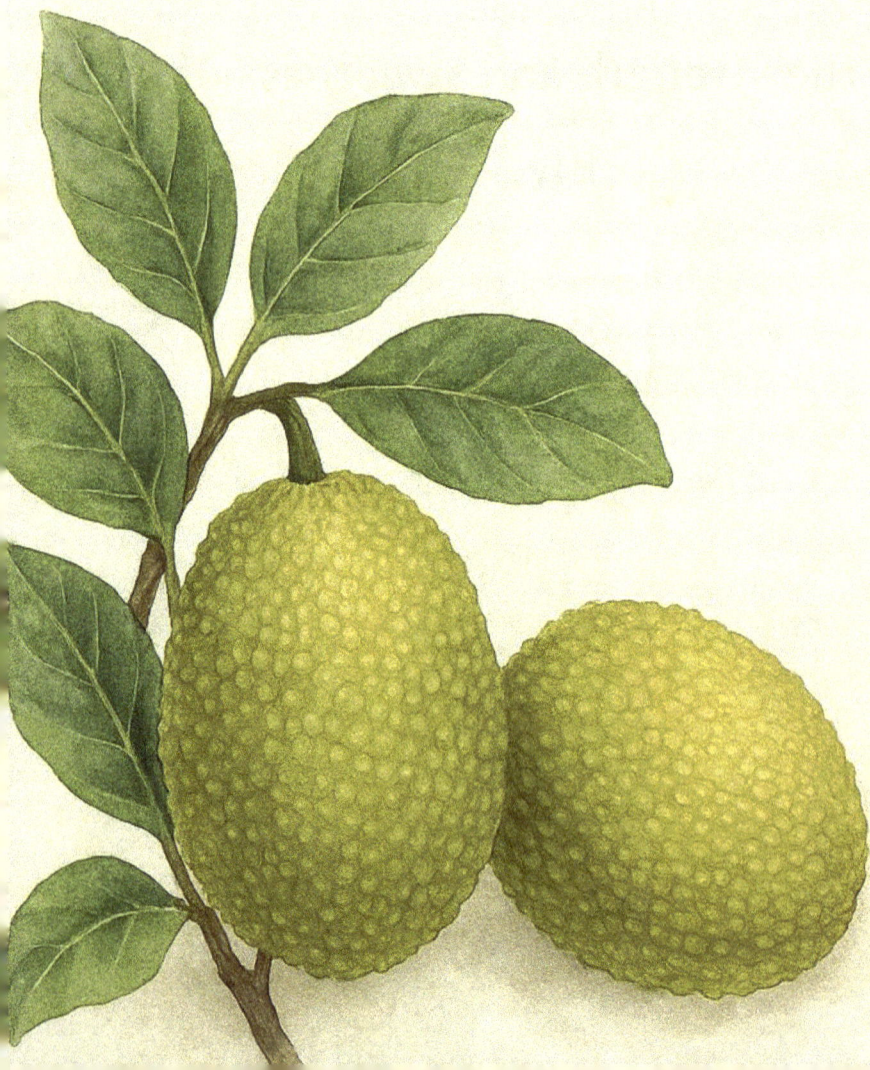

It is said that jackfruit grew in the ashrams of warriors and yogis—offering them energy, strength, and digestive support. Symbolically, jackfruit represents inner strength, hidden potential, and transformation.

## JACKFRUIT TEACHES:

- Your true sweetness is protected by your trials
- What is difficult to access often carries great value
- Nourishment sometimes requires effort, but brings deep rewards

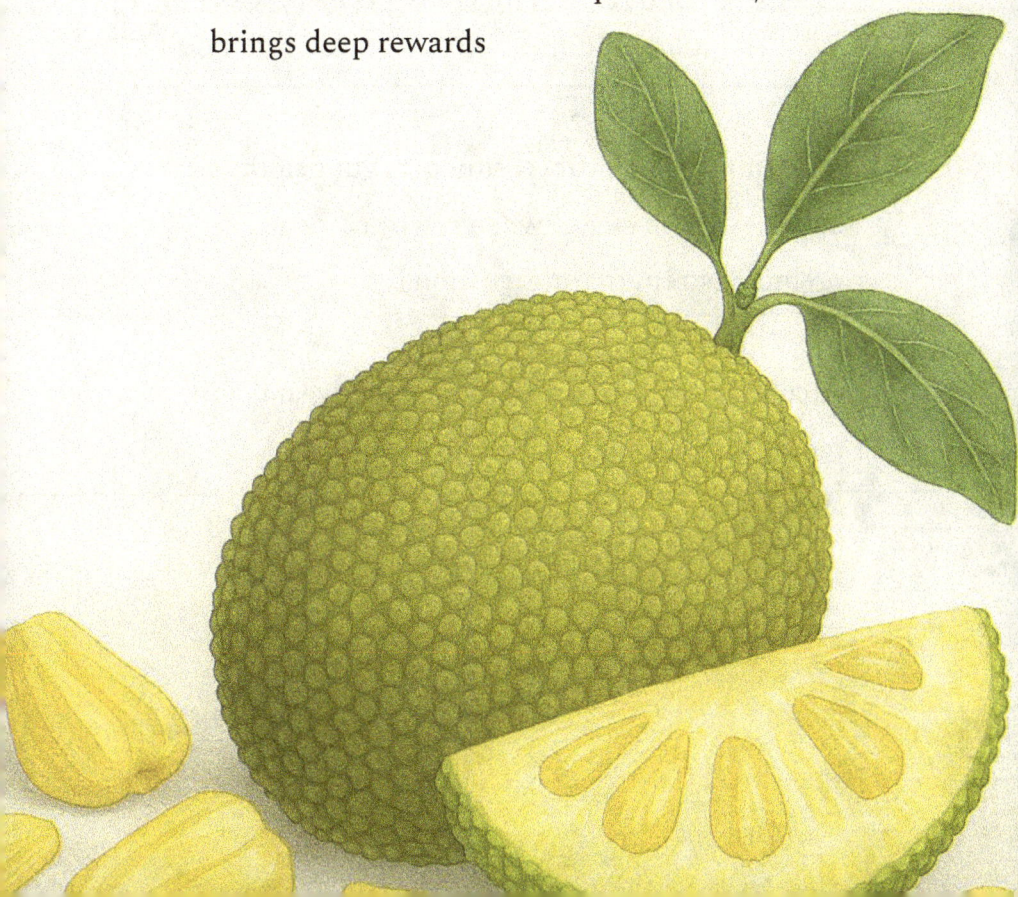

## NUTRITIONAL WHOLENESS OF JACKFRUIT

| Parts | Benefits | Uses |
|-------|----------|------|
| Raw Flesh | Low calorie, high fiber, B-complex vitamins | Curries, sabzi, tacos (meat substitute) |
| Ripe Flesh | Rich in natural sugars, Vitamin C, antioxidants | Eaten as fruit, desserts |
| Seeds | High in protein, zinc, magnesium | Boiled, roasted, made into flour |

Jackfruit is rich in fiber, supports gut health, balances blood sugar (when raw), and provides prebiotic strength for digestion.

Excellent for growing children, elderly, and anyone recovering from fatigue or weakness.

# EASY RECIPES & RITUALS WITH JACKFRUIT

### 1. Kathal Masala Curry (Raw Jackfruit)

Steam jackfruit chunks, sauté with mustard oil, ginger-garlic paste, onions, turmeric, garam masala.
Hearty and grounding—great for Vata and Kapha balance.

### 2. Ripe Jackfruit Chaat

Mix chopped ripe jackfruit with black salt, lemon juice, mint, and a dash of chili.
Uplifting and cooling—great digestive appetizer.

### 3. Jackfruit Seed Sabzi

Boil seeds, peel the outer layer, and cook with cumin, hing, tomato, and green chili.
Strengthens reproductive system and boosts stamina.

### 4. Jackfruit Stew with Coconut Milk

Use raw jackfruit in a South Indian-style stew with curry leaves, turmeric, and coconut milk.
Ideal for gut healing and nourishment during recovery.

## SPIRITUAL PRACTICES

- Meditate on the hidden sweetness of jackfruit: "May I honor my own layers and find strength in my softness."
- Offer the first fruit of the season to your home deity with gratitude: "Thank you for the strength to grow through my thorns."

## WHY JACKFRUIT DESERVES A PLACE ON YOUR PLATE

☑ One of India's most undervalued superfoods
☑ Grows abundantly in tropical regions—easy to cultivate and store
☑ Versatile in sweet, savory, raw, or cooked forms
☑ A sustainable alternative to meat—rich in fiber, low in cost

# CURRY LEAVES

## THE IRON-RICH WHISPER OF HEALING

"Small in size, grand in grace. A silent healer in every Indian kitchen."

## METAPHYSICAL STORY: THE LEAF OF QUIET STRENGTH

There's an old saying in the South: "If turmeric is the queen of spice, curry leaf is her whispering sage." Once, in a Himalayan ashram, a healer prayed for a plant that could help the poor stay nourished even without fancy meals. From that intention, Kadi Patta, or Curry Leaf, was born.

This humble leaf didn't shout for attention—it simply slipped into every meal, releasing its aroma and magic. Often discarded after cooking, the curry leaf became a symbol of quiet service, sacrificial healing, and hidden nourishment.

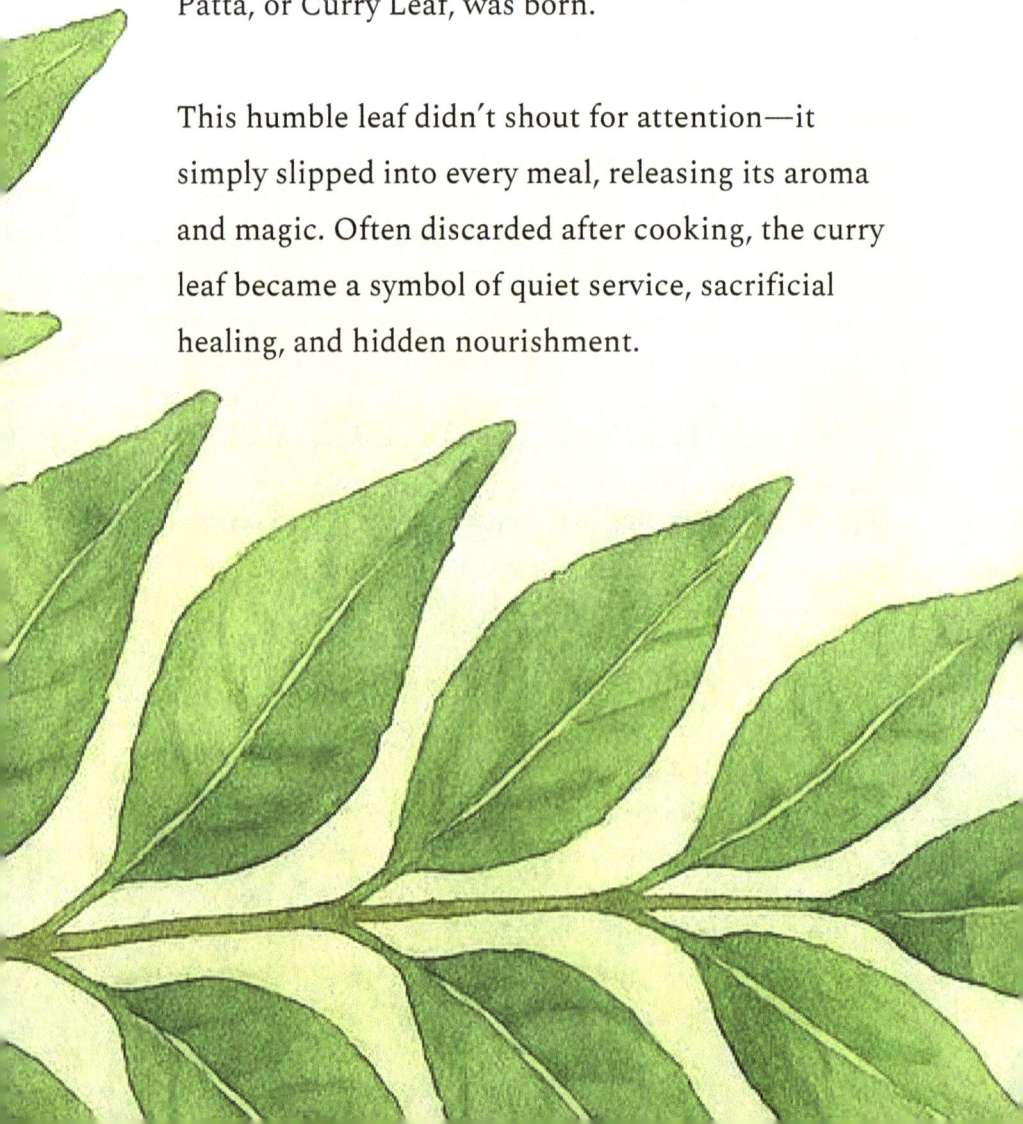

## CURRY LEAF TEACHES:

- You don't need to be loud to be powerful
- Serving others silently is its own form of medicine
- True nourishment often goes unnoticed, but it is vital

## NUTRITIONAL BRILLIANCE OF CURRY LEAF

Though tiny, curry leaves are packed with nutrition that deeply supports blood, bones, and digestion:

| Benefits | Uses |
| --- | --- |
| Iron & Folate | Helps in treating anemia naturally |
| Calcium & Phosphorus | Bone health and cell repair |
| Antioxidants | Reduce oxidative stress and protect organs |
| Essential Oils | Improve digestion, fight bacteria |

Curry Leaf supports hair growth, regulates blood sugar, boosts gut health, and improves eye function.

Especially beneficial for women, children, and anyone with chronic fatigue or dull skin.

## HEALING RECIPES WITH CURRY LEAVES

### 1. Curry Leaf Chutney

Grind curry leaves with roasted chana dal, garlic, green chili, lemon, and salt.

Pair with idli, dosa, or rice for iron-rich flavor.

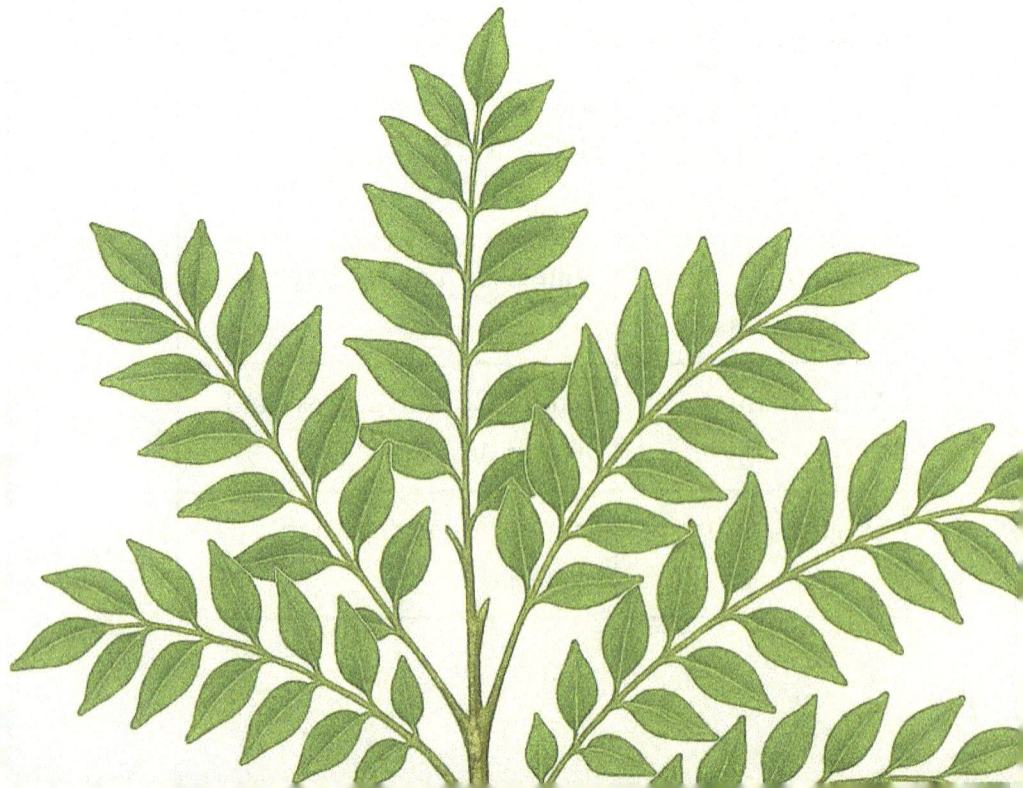

## 2. Curry Leaf Kadha (Tea for Digestion & Hair)

Boil curry leaves with cumin, ajwain, ginger, and a pinch of jaggery. Sip warm.

Excellent for post-meal detox and hair nourishment.

## 3. Curry Leaf Tempering (Tadka)

Add fresh curry leaves to hot ghee or oil with mustard seeds and hing.

Use on dals, sabzis, and khichdi for enhanced flavor and nutrient absorption.

## 4. Curry Leaf Oil for Hair Growth

Infuse coconut oil with curry leaves and fenugreek. Massage weekly.

Ancient formula for thick, shiny hair and cooling the scalp.

## SPIRITUAL PRACTICES

- Collect curry leaves with reverence and never waste them.

- While cooking, say mentally: "As I stir you into this food, let silent healing spread to all who eat."
- Place a small bowl of fresh curry leaves near your kitchen altar or stove as a symbol of sacred nourishment.

## WHY CURRY LEAVES BELONG IN YOUR DAILY LIFE

✅ Grows easily at home—pot or garden

✅ Used in traditional formulations for blood, liver, and skin

✅ Supports long-term vitality without cost

✅ Adds flavor and function to every meal

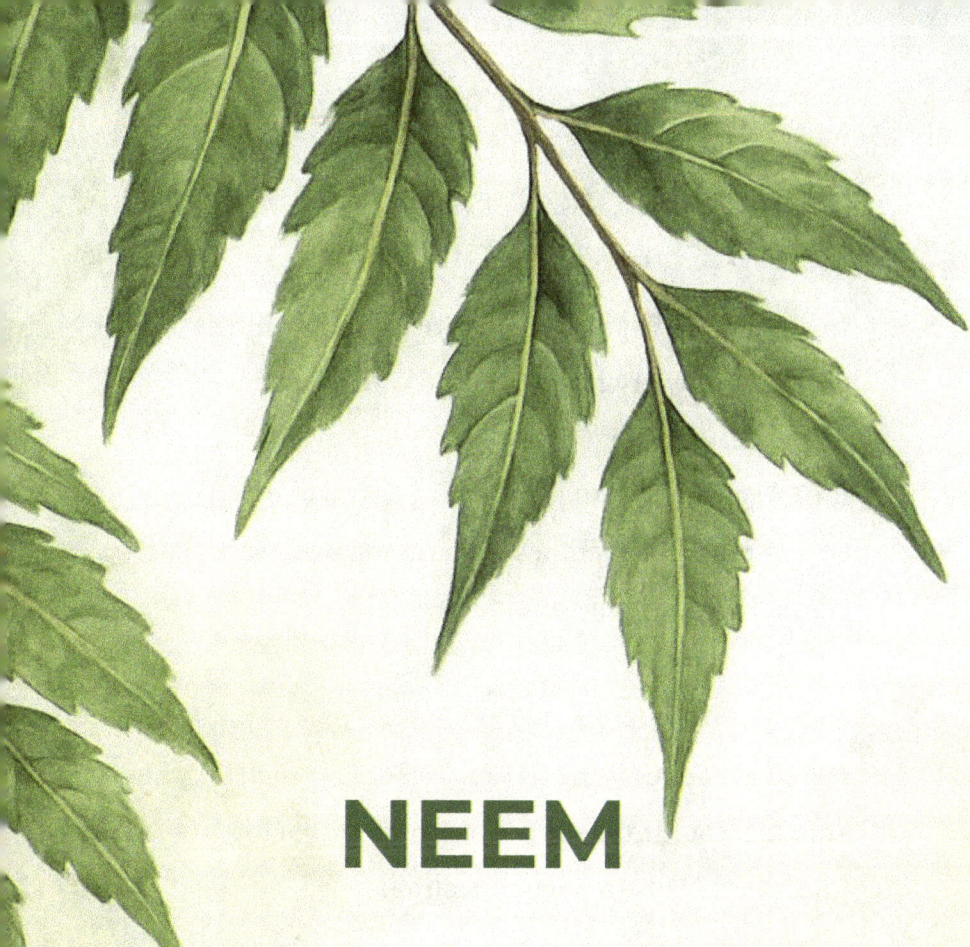

# NEEM

"Bitter is the taste of truth, and
from it springs lasting health."

## METAPHYSICAL STORY: THE SACRED SENTINEL OF THE THRESHOLD

In ancient India, neem trees were planted at the entrance of every home, temple, and village well. The elders believed that neem didn't just purify the air— it protected the soul. It was said that when evil spirits roamed, neem leaves hung on doorways warded off darkness and disease alike.

Neem came to be known as "Sarva Roga Nivarini" – the one that cures all ailments. Not just physical, but spiritual too. It taught people that embracing life's bitterness leads to deeper healing.

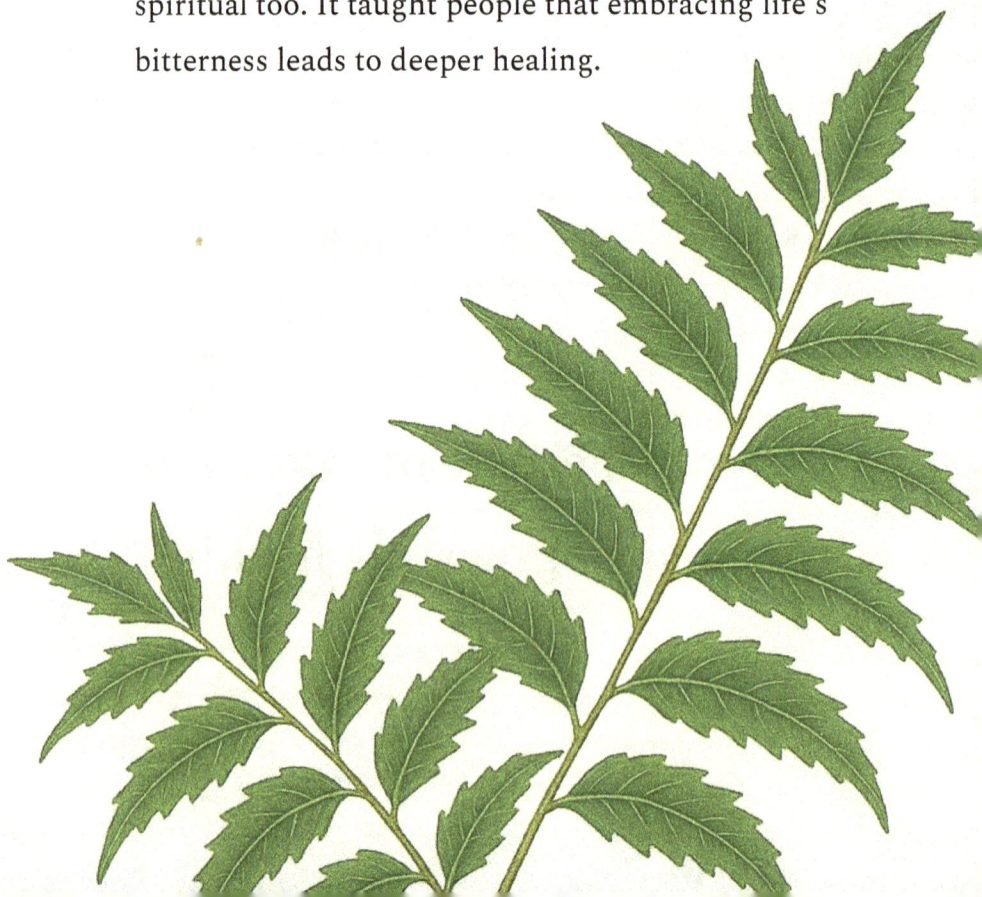

## NEEM TEACHES:

- Cleansing is the first step to transformation
- Healing isn't always sweet—it is deep, purifying, and sometimes uncomfortable
- Protect what you love by first purifying your own mind and space

## NUTRITIONAL BRILLIANCE OF NEEM

| Part Used | Benefits |
|---|---|
| Leaves | Blood purification, skin detox, anti-parasitic |
| Neem Oil | Anti-fungal, hair and scalp treatment, oral care |
| Bark Powder | Anti-diabetic, immune-boosting |
| Flowers | Liver tonic, menstrual balance |

Highly effective for acne, eczema, fungal infections, digestive parasites, and blood sugar control.

In Traditional medicine neem is classified as tikta (bitter) and kashaya (astringent) – both essential for detox and immune balance.

## EASY RECIPES & CLEANSING RITUALS WITH NEEM

### 1. Neem Leaf Detox Water

Boil a few neem leaves in water. Let it cool, and sip small amounts daily.

Cleanses liver, purifies blood, improves digestion.

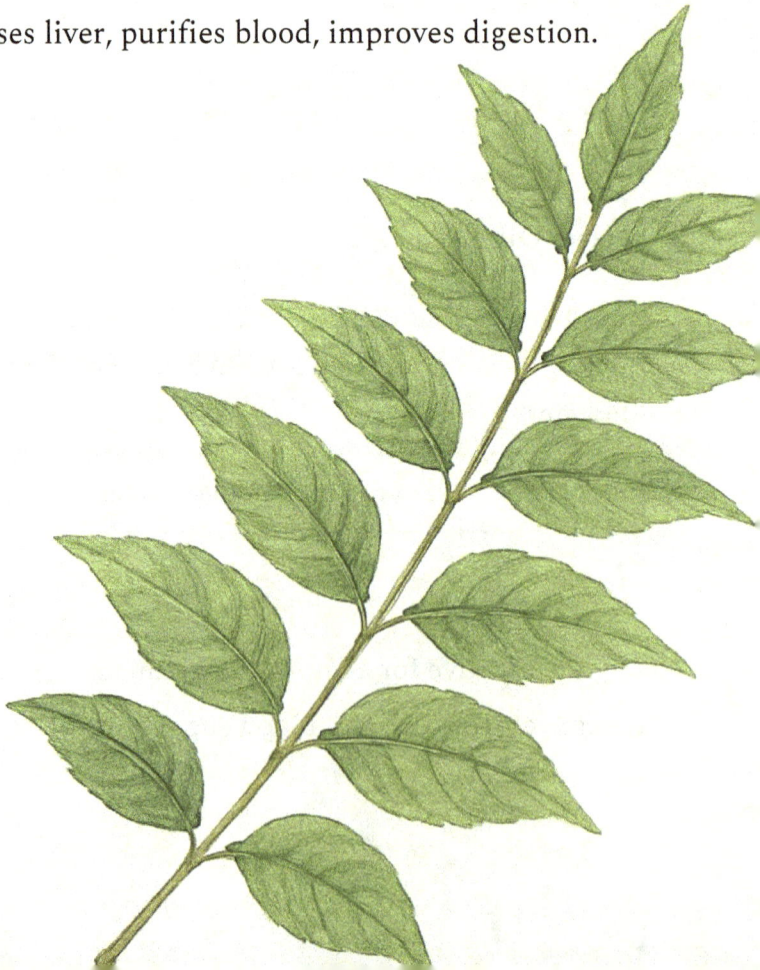

### 2. Neem Paste for Skin

Grind fresh neem leaves into a paste. Apply to face/body as a mask.

Clears acne, rashes, and deeply detoxifies pores.


### 3. Neem Oil Hair Treatment

Warm neem oil (mixed with coconut oil) and massage into scalp. Leave overnight.

Kills dandruff-causing microbes and supports hair growth.


### 4. Neem Flower Rasam (Traditional Tamil Detox Soup)

Cook neem flowers with tamarind, black pepper, and cumin.

A potent liver cleanser and digestive bitter—ideal during spring cleansing or after feasts.


## SPIRITUAL PRACTICES

- Hang neem leaves on your doorway on Amavasya (New Moon) to clear stagnant energy

- Burn dried neem leaves with camphor as natural incense to cleanse home energetically
- Say this prayer when consuming neem: "Let the bitterness I accept today dissolve all illusions and restore my inner purity."

## WHY NEEM IS SACRED AND ESSENTIAL

✅ Grows abundantly across India—zero maintenance

✅ Replaces many chemical medicines and cosmetic treatments

✅ Sacred in Indian rituals and healing since Vedic

✅ Deeply grounding, protective, and cleansing—both physically and energetically

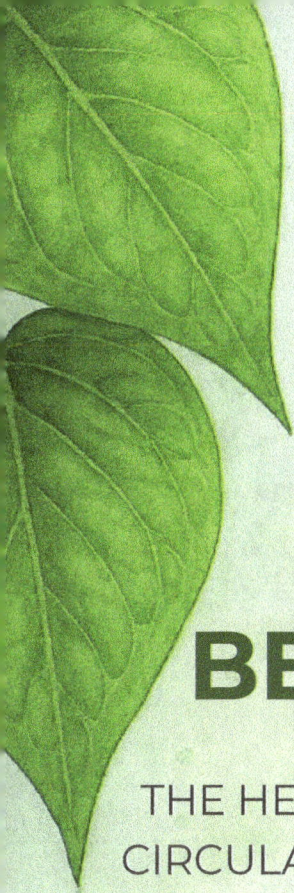

# BETEL LEAF

## THE HEART-SHAPED HEALER OF CIRCULATION AND CELEBRATION

"Where there is love, there is circulation—of life, breath, joy, and devotion."

## METAPHYSICAL STORY: THE LEAF OF CONNECTION

In Indian tradition, betel leaf (Paan) is not just a flavor or digestive—it is an offering of respect and love. Used in weddings, prayers, and festive occasions, the leaf is a symbol of heartful presence, of auspicious beginnings and warm conclusions.

Ancient poets wrote that giving someone a betel leaf was like handing them a piece of your own heart— fragrant, vital, alive.

In temples, it is offered to deities along with turmeric and coconut, signifying the balance of heat, coolness, and sweetness in life.

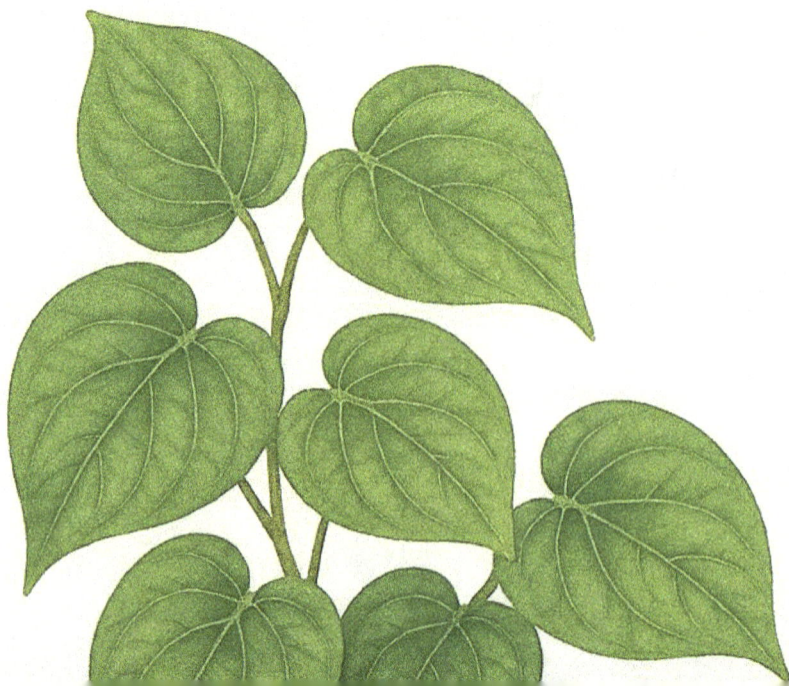

## BETEL TEACHES:

- Let your actions be heartfelt and fragrant
- True celebration arises when body and soul are both nourished
- Vitality flows where joy and ritual meet

## NUTRITIONAL & MEDICINAL PROPERTIES OF BETEL LEAF

Betel leaf is an aromatic stimulant, mild aphrodisiac, and natural digestive. It supports circulation, oral hygiene, and hormonal health, especially in women.

| Benefit | Explanation |
|---|---|
| Digestive Aid | Stimulates saliva and enzymes; soothes the gut |
| Circulation Booster | Improves blood flow and heart vitality |
| Antimicrobial | Fights oral bacteria and freshens breath |
| Mood Enhancer | Its aroma and essential oils can calm the mind |

# DAILY WAYS TO USE BETEL LEAF

### 1. Traditional Digestive Paan

Wrap a small piece of fennel, coconut, and cardamom inside a fresh betel leaf. Chew slowly after meals.
Supports digestion, sweetens breath, refreshes senses.

### 2. Betel Leaf Infusion (Herbal Tea)

Steep fresh betel leaves with tulsi and lemongrass. Boosts circulation, relieves bloating, and calms anxiety.

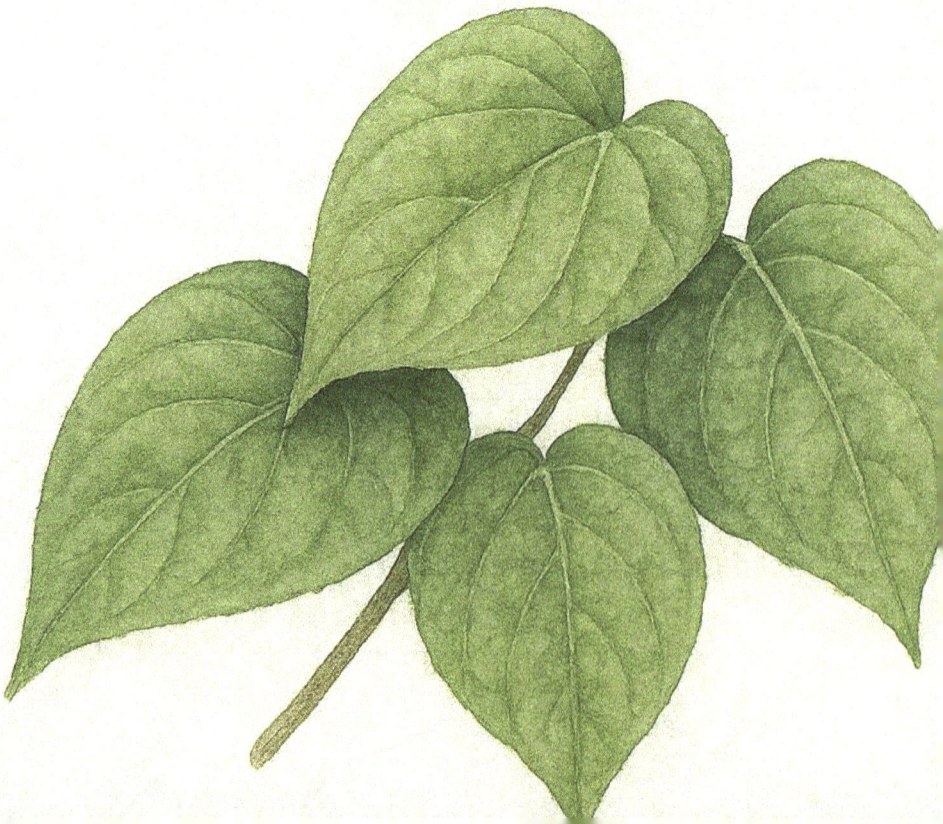

### 3. Betel in Facial Steam

Boil betel leaves in water and inhale steam.
Opens pores, clears nasal passages, improves blood flow to skin.

### 4. Topical Use for Pain Relief

Warm the leaf and apply to swollen joints or chest (during cough).
Relieves inflammation and encourages circulation.

## SPIRITUAL PRACTICES

- Offered to Goddess Lakshmi and Lord Ganesha during rituals
- Given to brides and grooms during marriage ceremonies for love
- Used in Navaratri and Diwali pujas as an auspicious herb of celebration and cleansing

## AFFIRMATION

"May love flow through my body like breath through a leaf—fragrant, alive, and healing."

## WHY BETEL LEAF BELONGS IN YOUR KITCHEN & ALTAR

✅ Common, affordable, and grown in most Indian homes or gardens

✅ Combines spiritual, sensual, and medicinal values

✅ Works on digestive, circulatory, and emotional health

✅ Encourages presence, celebration, and sacred connection

# TULSI

## THE QUEEN OF SACRED IMMUNITY

"In every home where Tulsi lives, the breath of health, grace, and divine protection lingers."

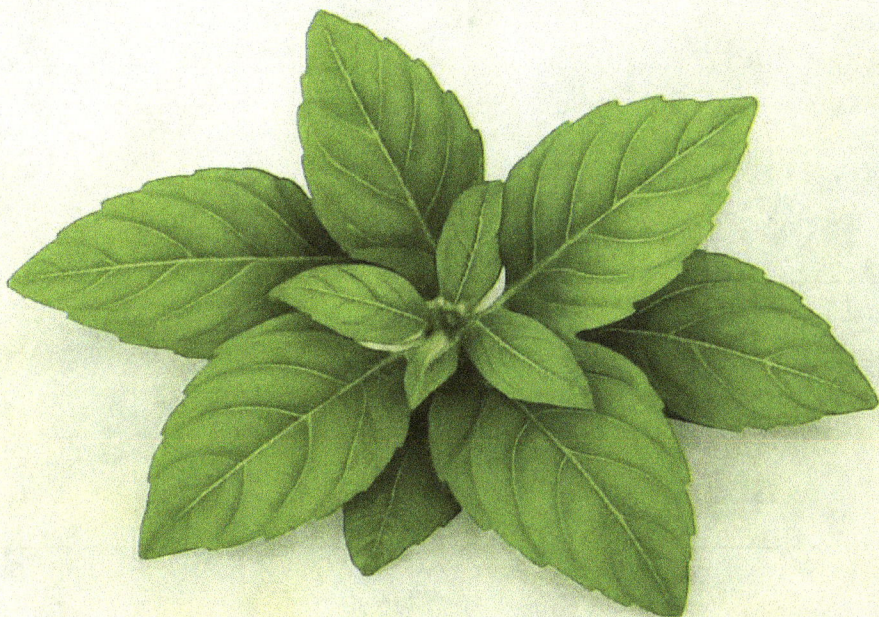

## METAPHYSICAL STORY

According to ancient lore, Tulsi was once a devoted woman named Vrinda, whose unwavering faith transformed her into a sacred plant. Lord Vishnu blessed her with immortality as Tulsi Devi, saying she would always reside in homes that honor her, purify spaces with her presence, and awaken spiritual consciousness.

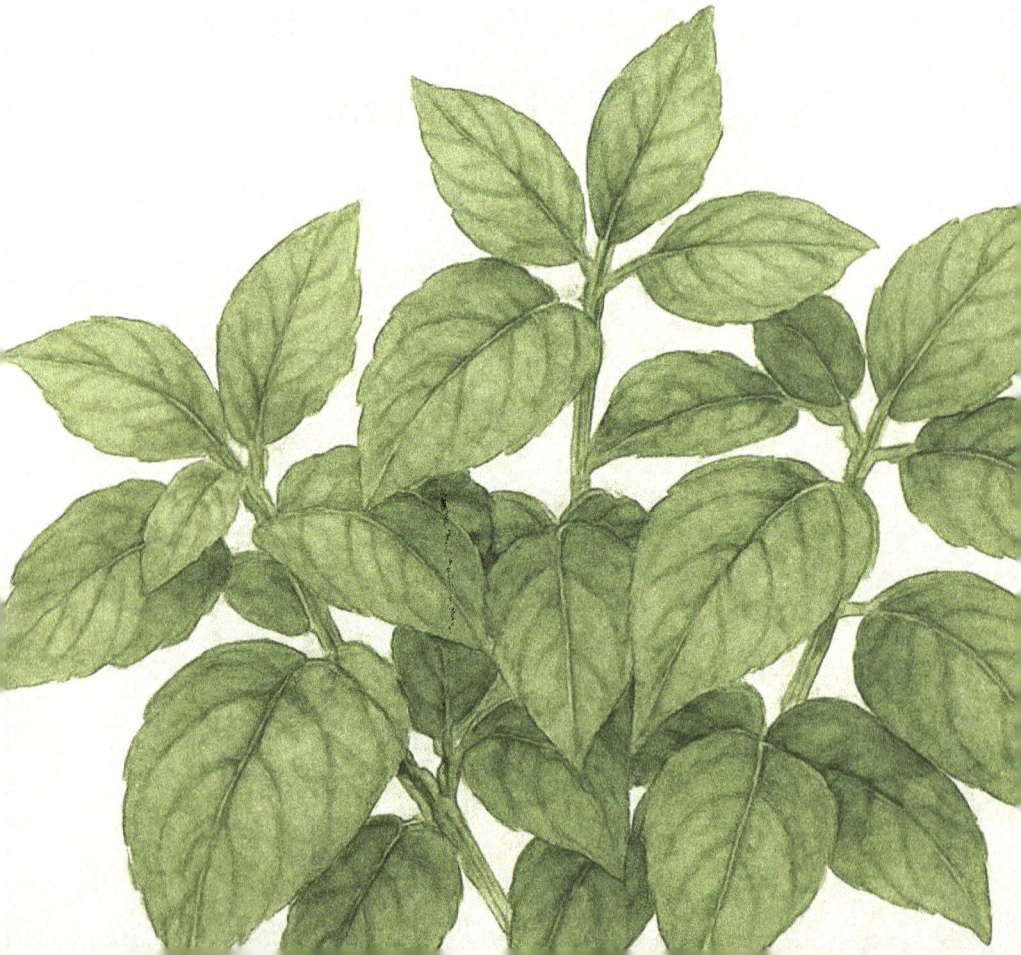

She stands for unshakable devotion, resilience, and selfless love—and imparts the same to those who consume her essence.

Tulsi (Holy Basil) is not just a plant—it's a living goddess. Found at the heart of courtyards and altars across India, Tulsi is worshipped, sipped, inhaled, and applied—for healing body, mind, and soul.

## UNIQUE NUTRITIONAL & MEDICINAL QUALITIES

- Adaptogenic: Balances cortisol and reduces stress
- Immunomodulatory: Strengthens immune responses
- Antibacterial, antifungal, antiviral
- Relieves respiratory conditions, fever, headaches
- Rich in vitamin C, iron, zinc, and essential oils

## DAILY RITUALS & RECIPES WITH TULSI LEAF

### 1. Tulsi Tea for Immunity

Boil fresh tulsi leaves with crushed ginger and black pepper.

Supports immunity, relieves cold and stress.

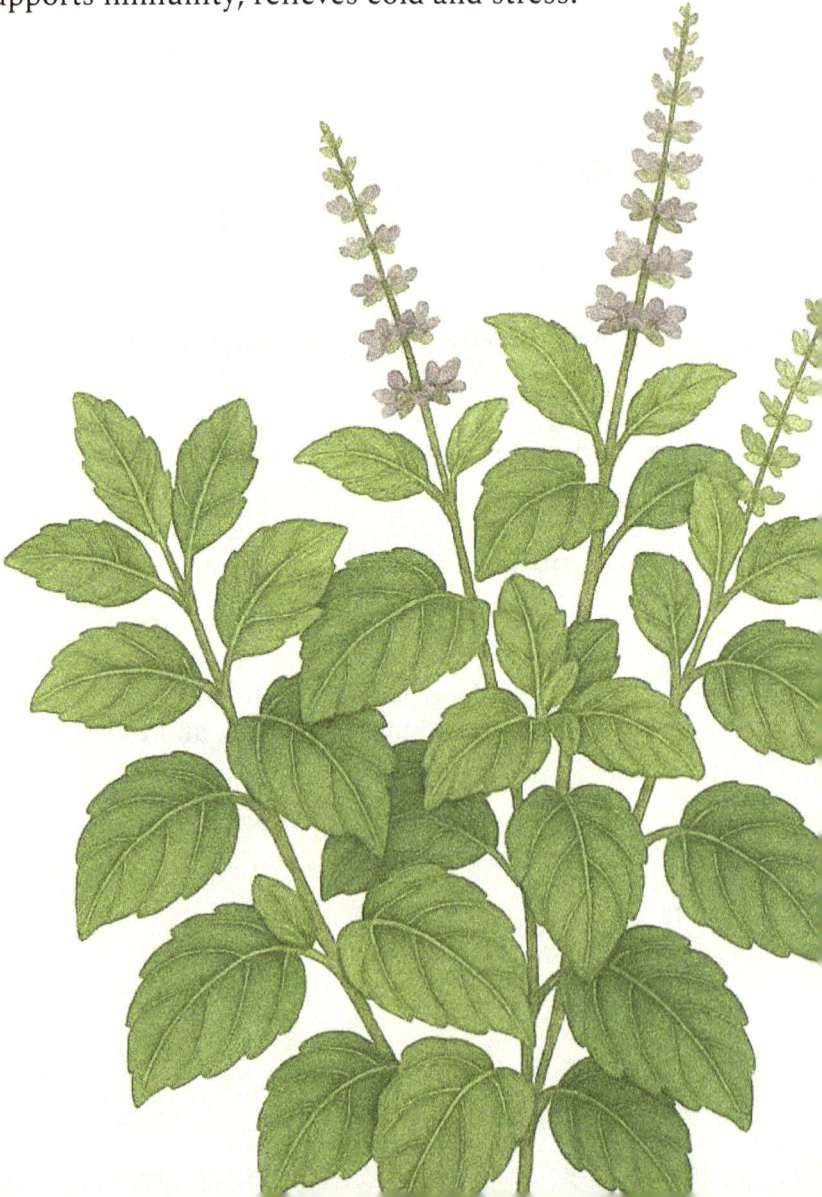

### 2. Tulsi Steam Inhalation

Add tulsi leaves to boiling water. Inhale with a towel over your head.

Clears sinuses, relieves headaches, and uplifts energy.

### 3. Tulsi Face Tonic

Steep tulsi in rose water. Spray as a cooling facial mist.

Soothes acne, refreshes and purifies skin.

### 4. Raw Tulsi Leaf Chewing

Chew 2–3 fresh leaves on an empty stomach.

Balances metabolism, clears toxins, improves breath.

## SPIRITUAL PRACTICES

- Place a Tulsi plant in the north or east direction of your home
- Offer water to Tulsi at sunrise with a prayer
- Light a ghee lamp near Tulsi in the evening— invites clarity and peace

- Tulsi Vivah (ritual marriage of Tulsi and Vishnu) is celebrated in Kartik month

## AFFIRMATION

"With every breath of Tulsi, I invite sacred immunity, divine devotion, and inner peace."

## WHY TULSI IS ESSENTIAL IN DAILY LIFE

✅ Combines spiritual purity and practical healing

✅ Grows easily in pots, balconies, and home gardens

✅ Deeply protective, purifying, and calming

✅ Elevates both immunity and consciousness

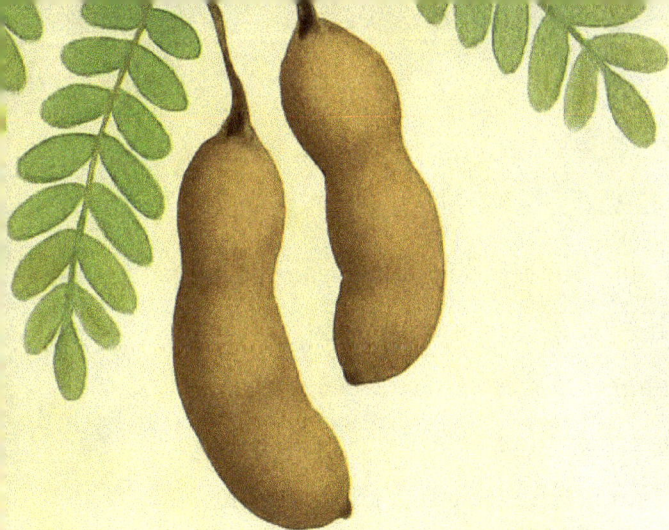

# TAMARIND

## THE TANGY TRANSFORMER OF METABOLISM

"Tangy to the tongue, cleansing to the gut, cooling to the fire— Tamarind is the alchemist of digestion."

## METAPHYSICAL STORY

In folk traditions, Tamarind trees are said to house powerful spirits—sometimes protectors, sometimes tricksters. Villagers respect these trees with quiet reverence. The tree's tangy pods represent life's bittersweet lessons: what purifies may first shock you. What cleanses may not always taste sweet.

In South Indian rituals, tamarind water is used to clean sacred idols—believing it washes away ego, excess, and energetic impurities.

Tamarind, or Imli, is the flavorful medicine hidden in almost every Indian kitchen. A puckering burst of sourness with cooling depth, Tamarind is more than a spice—it's a transformer of inner heat, a balancer of bile, and a digestive reset button.

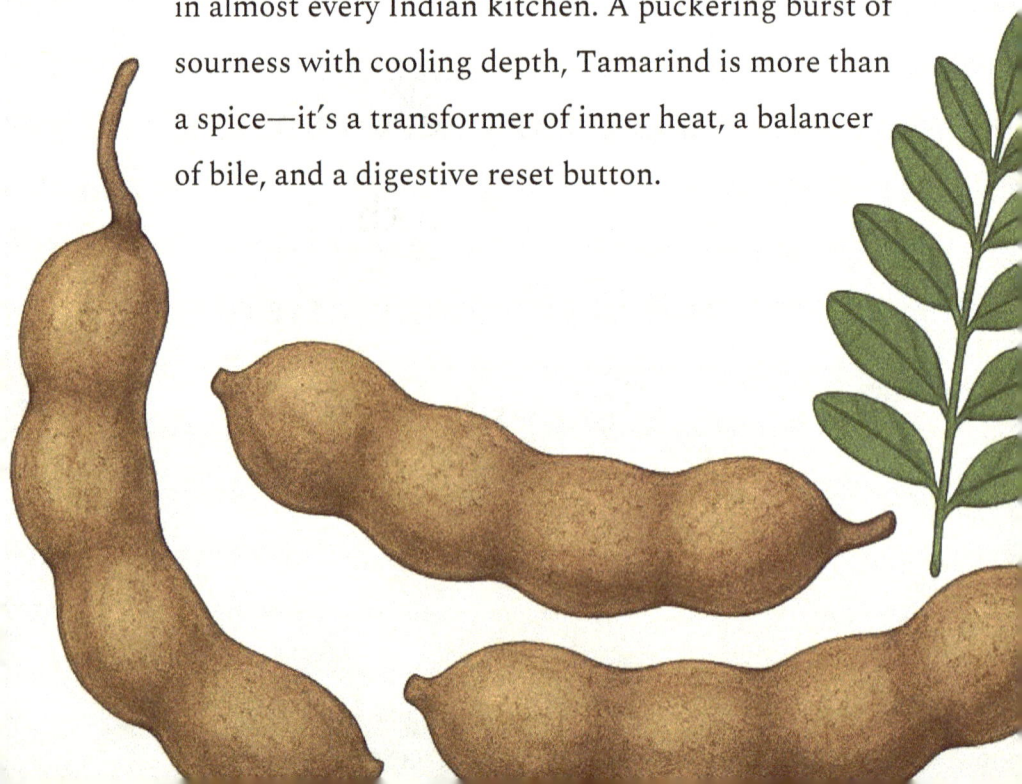

## NUTRITIONAL & HEALING PROPERTIES

- Rich in tartaric acid, potassium, magnesium, and iron
- Excellent for cleansing the liver and bile ducts
- Reduces inflammation and fights parasites
- Acts as a natural laxative and digestive stimulant
- Balances pitta dosha by cooling excess internal heat

## SIMPLE RECIPES & HEALING USES OF TAMARIND

### 1. Tamarind Digestive Water

Soak tamarind pulp in warm water. Add cumin and a pinch of rock salt.
Drink before meals to stimulate digestion and reduce bloating.

## 2. Tamarind Rasam

Cook tamarind pulp with black pepper, garlic, and mustard seeds.

A light detoxifying soup that cools and balances metabolism.

## 3. Imli Chutney for Cooling Heat

Blend tamarind with jaggery, ginger, and black salt.

Acts as a post-meal digestive and helps curb sugar cravings.

## 4. Tamarind Hair Rinse

Boil tamarind in water, cool, and use as a hair rinse.

Removes dandruff and balances scalp heat.

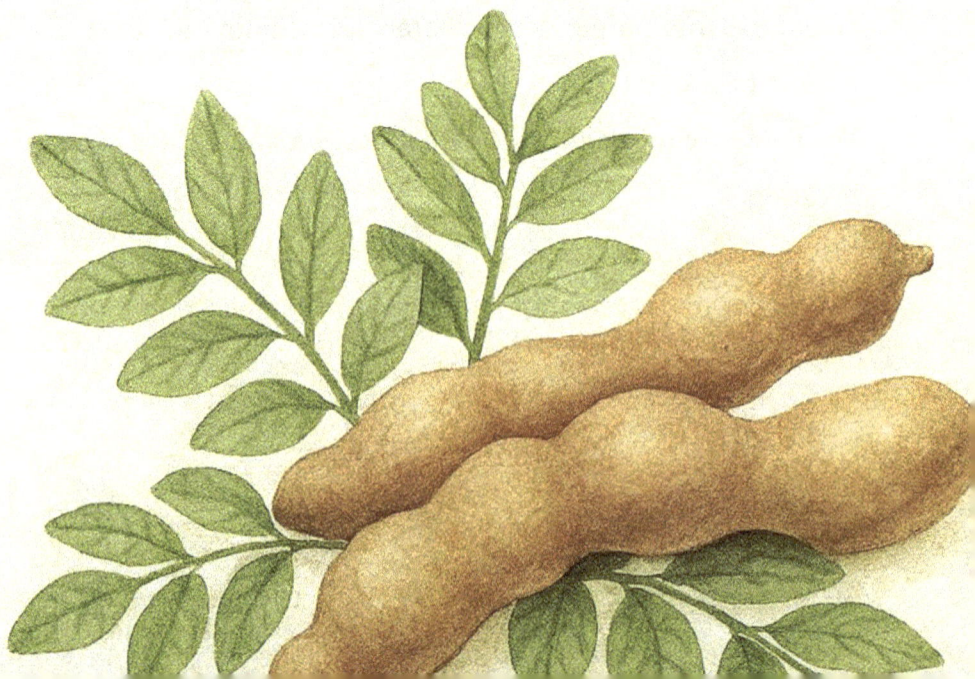

## SPIRITUAL PRACTICES

- Use tamarind water to cleanse kitchen altars or sacred objects
- Offer tamarind to Devi or Bhairava to clear intense energies
- Recite this mantra before consuming: "May the tang that touches my tongue awaken clarity in my belly and fire in my transformation."

## AFFIRMATION

"Let the tang of life cleanse my mind, clear my body, and stir my soul's truth."

## WHY TAMARIND IS A MUST-HAVE

☑ Used in Ayurvedic formulas for digestion and heat disorders

☑ Inexpensive, long-shelf-life, and used in both raw and cooked forms

☑ Can replace acidic vinegars or commercial souring agents

☑ Emotionally grounding and spiritually purifying

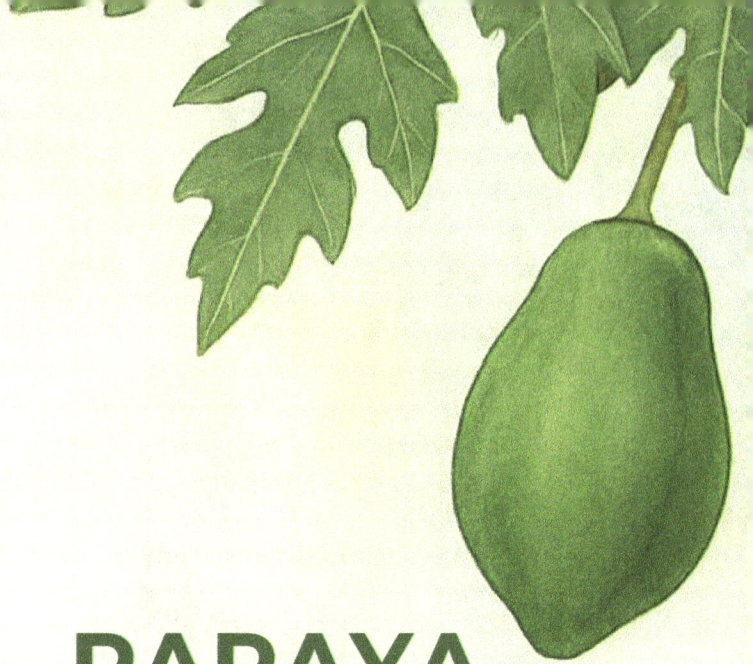

# PAPAYA

## THE GENTLE HEALER OF THE GUT & SKIN

"Soft to hold, strong in healing—Papaya is the fruit that listens to your stomach and whispers to your skin."

## METAPHYSICAL STORY

In ancient Indian folklore, papaya trees were believed to purify the energy of the home. Planted near the kitchen or back door, they symbolized digestive clarity and feminine healing.

Some healers whispered that papaya trees bloom best where gentleness is honored—and their milky sap was said to carry the secret signature of maternal love and intuitive repair. It's a plant that heals by softening—not through fire, but through grace.

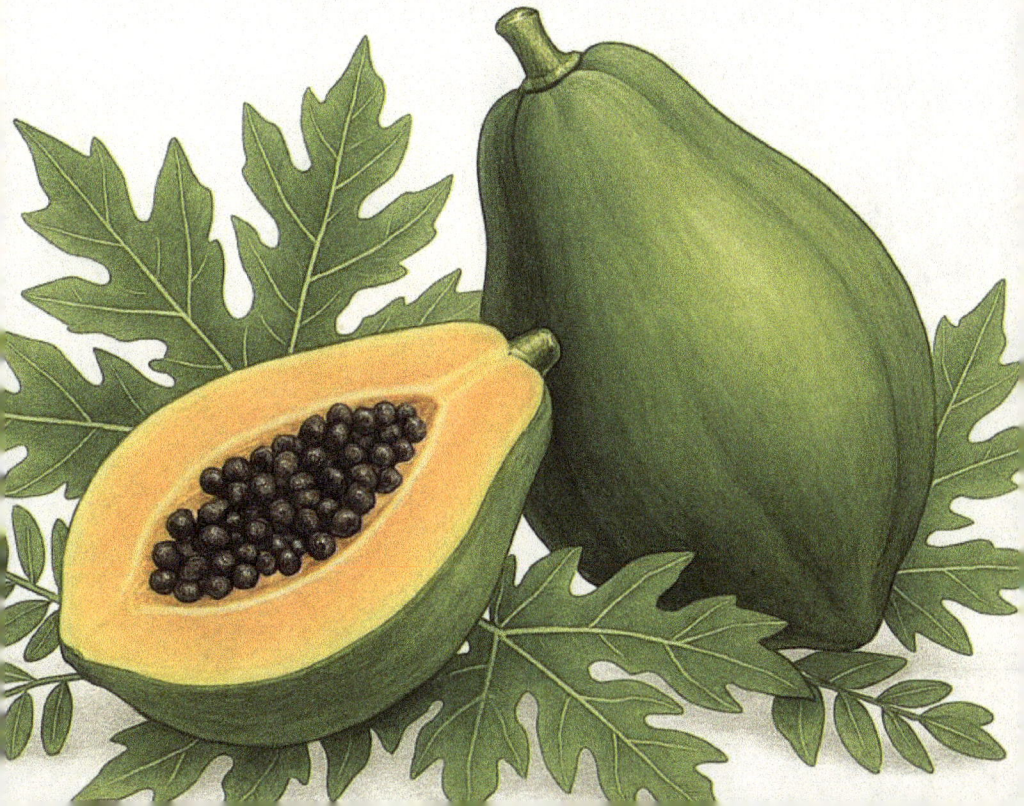

Papaya, known as "Erandakarkati" in Ayurveda, is the ultimate soother—gently digesting, detoxing, and rejuvenating from the inside out. A fruit that doesn't scream for attention but offers profound benefits for those who make space for softness and ease.

## NUTRITIONAL & HEALING PROPERTIES

- Rich in papain enzyme – supports protein digestion and soothes inflammation
- Excellent source of Vitamin C, A, and folate
- Supports skin regeneration, reduces acne and blemishes
- Aids bowel movement and relieves constipation and acidity
- Known for anti-parasitic and wound-healing effects

# EASY RECIPES & REMEDIES WITH PAPAYA

### 1. Papaya Breakfast Bowl

Blend ripe papaya with banana and lime juice. Add soaked seeds or nuts.

Soothes digestion, nourishes skin, and balances energy for the day.

### 2. Papaya Face Mask

Mash ripe papaya with honey and a pinch of turmeric. Apply to face.

Brightens skin, reduces pigmentation, and unclogs pores.

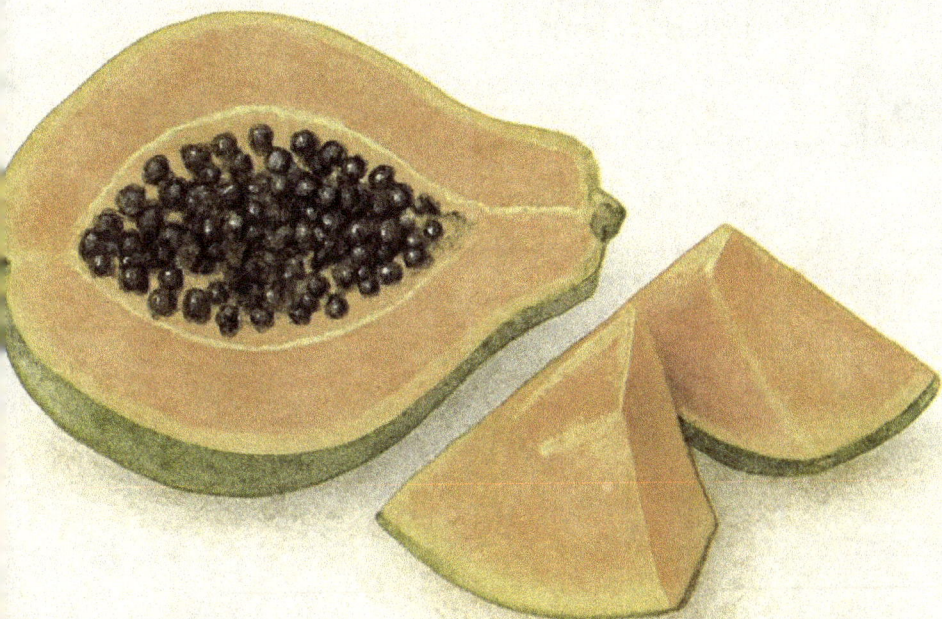

### 3. Unripe Papaya Curry (South Indian Style)

Cook green papaya with curry leaves, coconut, and mustard seeds.

A healing dish for gut strength and enzyme support.

### 4. Papaya Leaf Juice (Bitter but Potent)

Extract juice from young leaves, mix with a few drops of lemon.

Known to support blood platelet count and detoxify the liver.

## SPIRITUAL PRACTICES

- Offer papaya during Sankranti or spring rituals for renewal and cleansing
- Use papaya leaf in ritual baths for gentle release of emotional burdens
- Whisper this blessing before eating: "May this fruit soften my edges, digest my pain, and nourish my glow."

## AFFIRMATION

"With each bite, I receive kindness, clarity, and calm from the heart of the fruit."

## WHY PAPAYA BELONGS IN YOUR EVERYDAY HEALING

✅ Affordable and available all year in tropical climates

✅ Supports both digestive and skin health—a rare dual healer

✅ A gentle food for the elderly, children, and post-illness recovery

✅ Acts as a food-medicine when eaten raw, ripe, or cooked

# GINGER

## THE FIERY ROOT OF VITALITY

"From the deep womb of the Earth, Ginger rises like fire— awakening our digestion, circulation, and willpower."

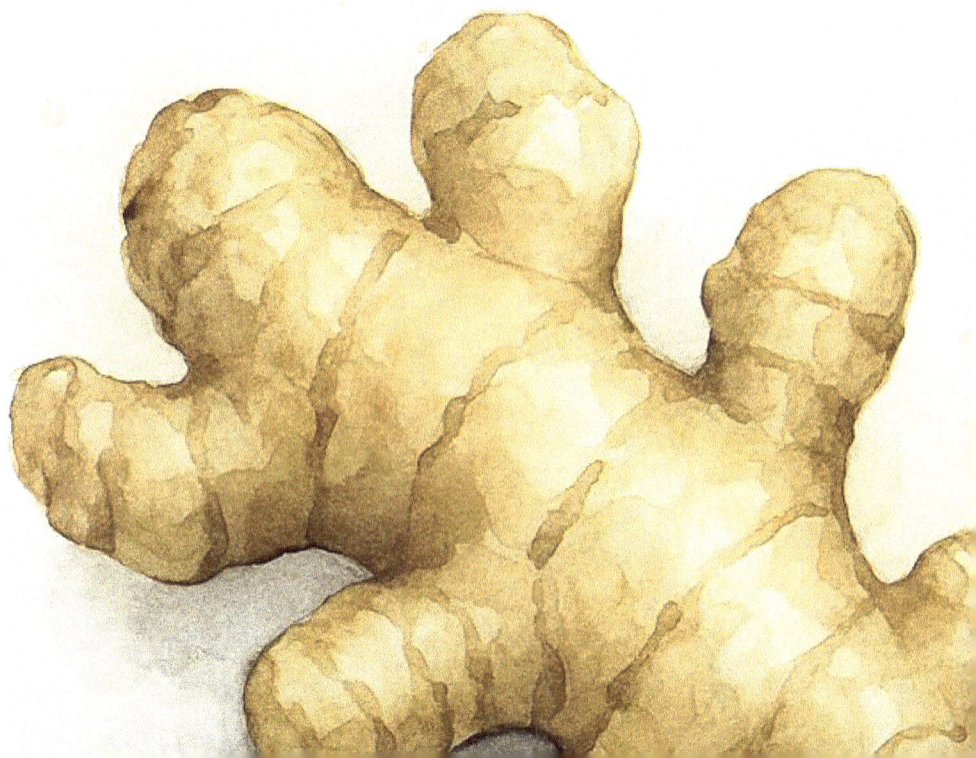

## METAPHYSICAL STORY

It is said in folk wisdom that ginger grew first where
Shakti's tears touched the soil—tears not of grief,
but of fierce compassion and awakening. Where
other herbs cool or cleanse, ginger ignites. In
Ayurveda, it's called Vishvabhesaj—"The Universal
Medicine."

Healers use ginger when someone is stuck: stuck in
digestion, stuck in sadness, stuck in stagnation. It is
the spark that brings warmth to cold bellies, tired
blood, and heavy hearts.

In every Indian kitchen, a humble root rests in a
corner—knobby, fragrant, and ancient. Ginger, or
Adrak, is not just a spice. It's a catalyst, a warrior, a
medicine, and a soul warmer. It activates whatever it
touches—be it a dish, a body, or a foggy morning
mind.

## NUTRITIONAL & HEALING PROPERTIES

- Boosts digestive fire (Agni) and relieves nausea, gas, and bloating
- Powerful anti-inflammatory—supports joint health and pain relief
- Enhances circulation and warms the body
- Fights cold, flu, and respiratory congestion
- Aids detoxification by promoting sweating and blood flow

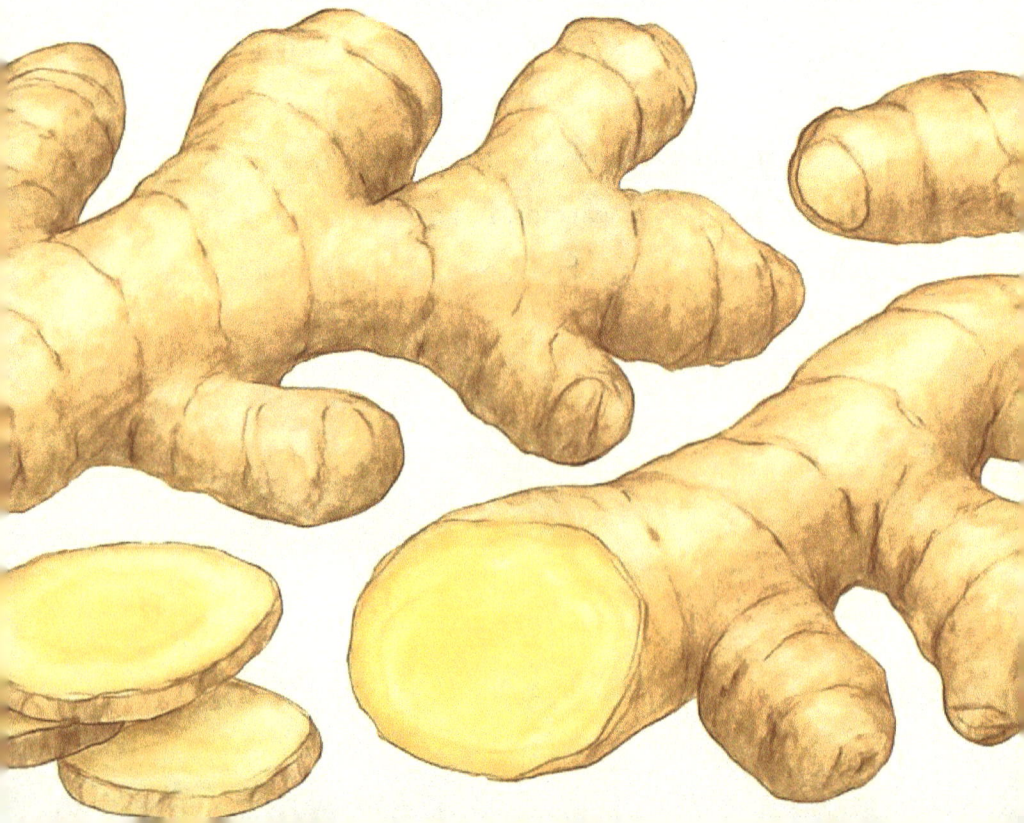

# EASY RECIPES & HEALING RITUALS WITH GINGER

### 1. Ginger-Lemon Morning Tea

Boil crushed ginger with water. Add fresh lemon juice and honey.

Kickstarts metabolism, cleanses the system, and strengthens immunity.

### 2. Ginger Compress

Wrap grated ginger in a cloth, steep in hot water, and apply to sore areas.

Relieves menstrual cramps, joint stiffness, and chest congestion.

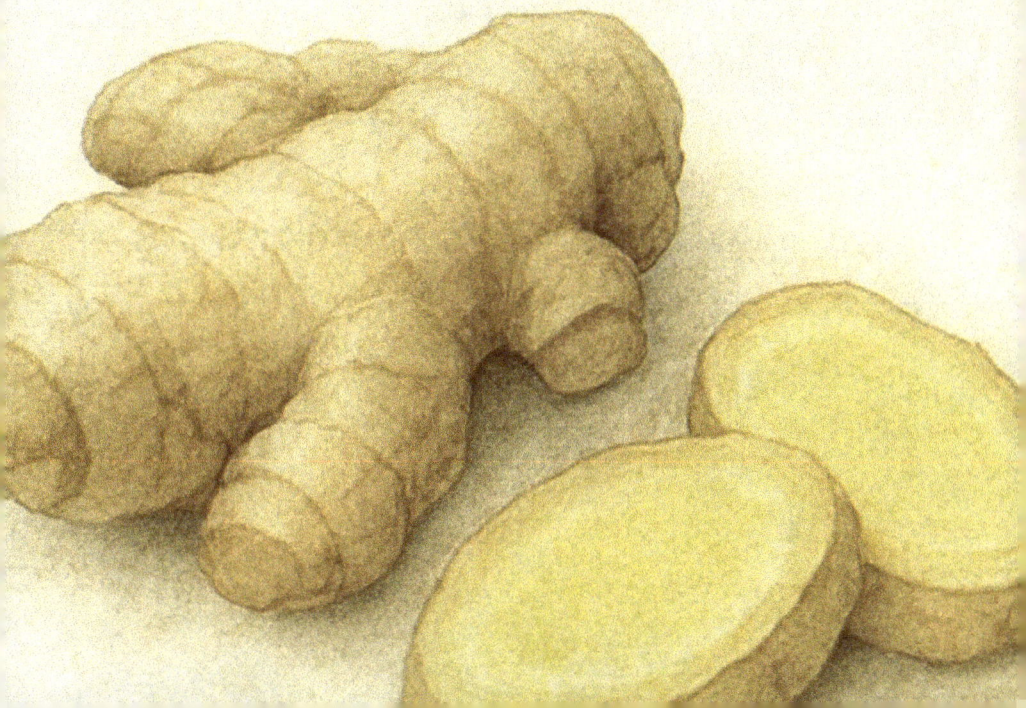

### 3. Adrak-Tulsi Kadha (Healing Decoction)

Simmer fresh ginger with tulsi, black pepper, and jaggery. Sip warm.
A classic Indian drink to fight infections and lift energy.

### 4. Ginger Stir Fry Tadka

Add fresh grated ginger to oil with mustard seeds before making curries or dals.
Infuses warmth and digestive strength into every dish.

## SPIRITUAL PRACTICES

- Offer dried ginger pieces in homam (fire offerings) to awaken inner clarity
- Rub ginger oil on soles before meditation to ground and energize
- Light a lamp near ginger plant or root during winter full moons for vitality
- Chant this while consuming ginger: "With this flame of earth, I awaken strength, clarity, and courage in every cell."

## AFFIRMATION

"I carry the fire of the Earth within me—steady, warm, and ready to transform."

## WHY GINGER IS YOUR KITCHEN'S ROOT GURU

- ✅ Affordable, grows easily even in a pot
- ✅ Can be used fresh, dried, or powdered—year-round support
- ✅ Enhances all systems: digestion, circulation, immunity, clarity
- ✅ Symbol of resilience, warmth, and energetic protection

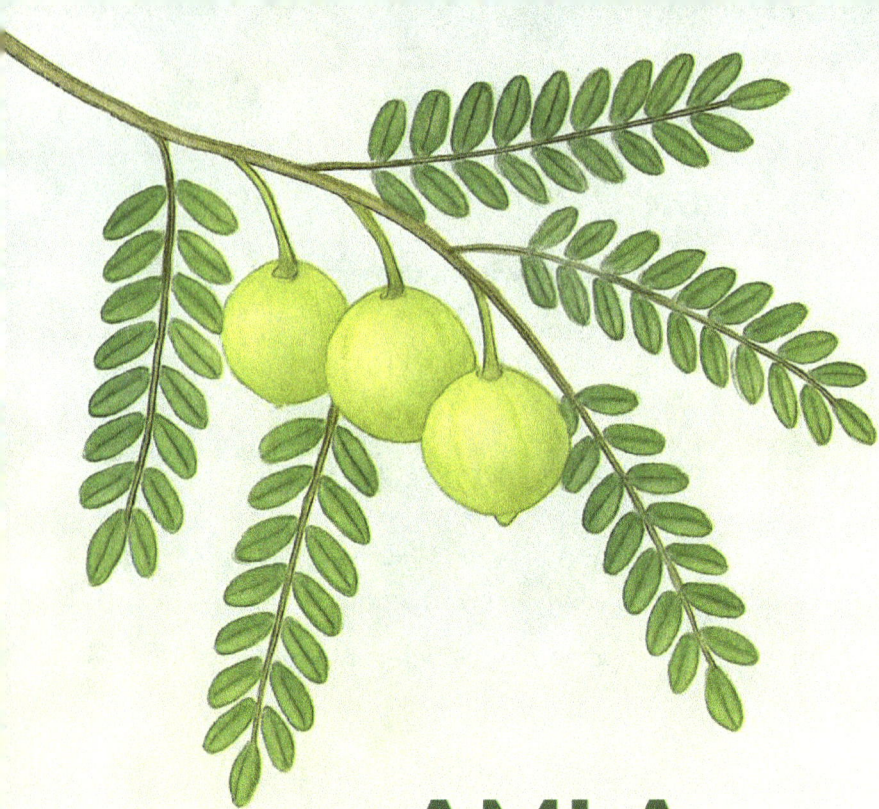

# AMLA

## THE RADIANT FRUIT OF IMMORTALITY

"Where light meets sourness,
life is renewed."

## METAPHYSICAL STORY

Ancient texts say that when the gods and demons churned the cosmic ocean (Samudra Manthan) for the nectar of immortality, Amla was born from the first drop of amrit that touched the Earth. That is why it is known as Divya-Phala—the divine fruit.

Just as the soul is unaging, Amla restores us to our original vitality—radiant, balanced, whole.

In the forests of India grows a modest green berry, round and sour—but inside it, a secret of longevity glows. Amla, or Indian Gooseberry, is not just a fruit. It is Ayurveda's elixir, a rasayana—a rare gift that nourishes, rebuilds, and protects the body at the deepest level.

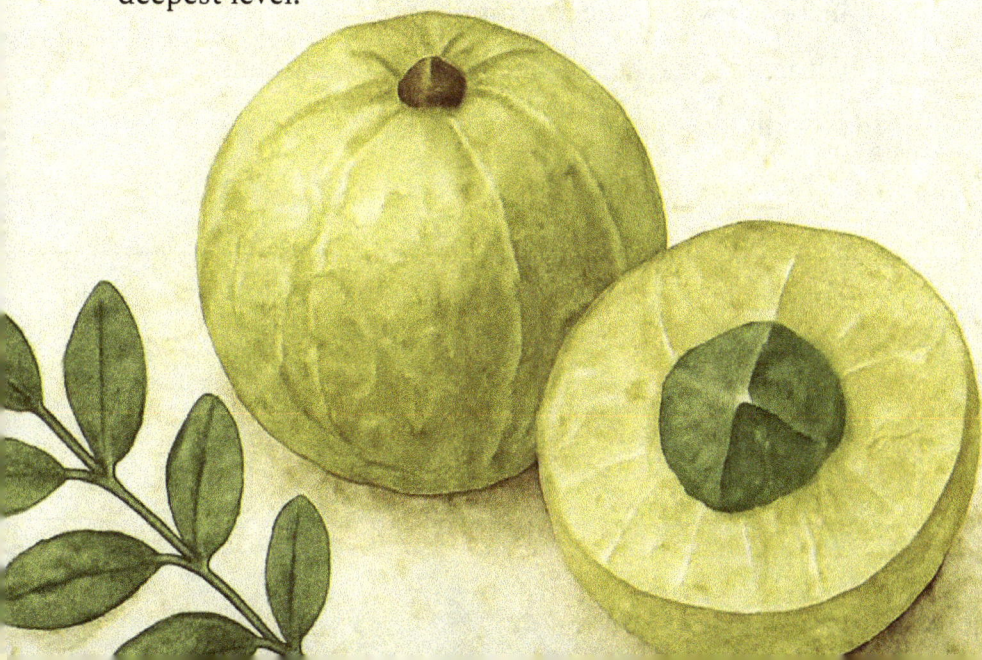

## NUTRITIONAL & HEALING PROPERTIES

- Richest natural source of Vitamin C—boosts immunity
- Balances all three doshas—vata, pitta, kapha
- Regenerates liver cells and blood tissue
- Enhances eye health, skin glow, and hair strength
- Supports mental clarity, memory, and emotional resilience

## EASY DAILY WAYS TO USE AMLA

### 1. Fresh Amla Juice

Blend amla with water, a pinch of black salt, and honey. Drink in the morning.
Cleanses liver, boosts energy, and strengthens digestion.

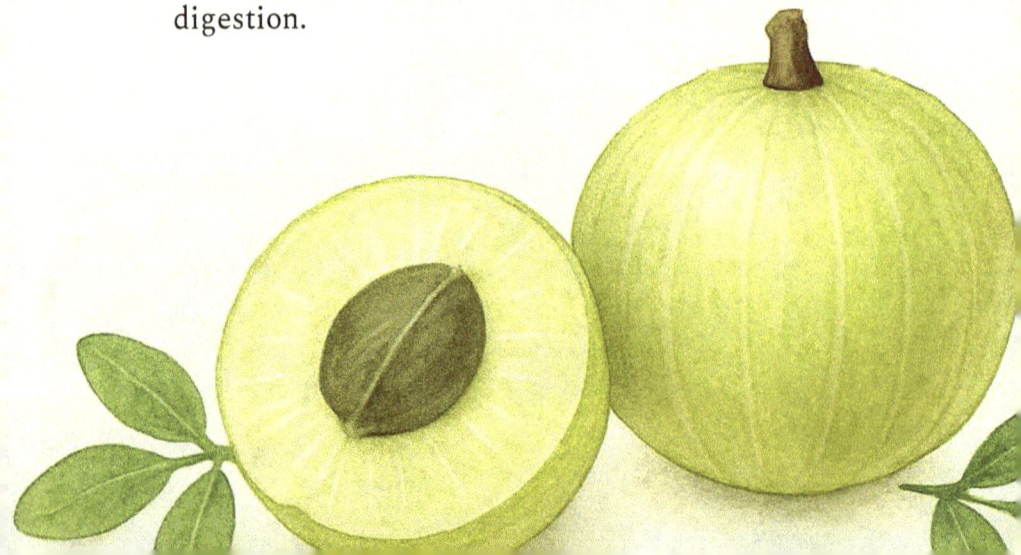

## 2. Triphala Powder at Night

Take a teaspoon of Triphala (which includes amla) with warm water before bed.
Gentle detox, promotes regular elimination and glowing skin.

## 3. Amla Chutney

Grind raw amla with coriander, ginger, and green chili.
A tangy immunity booster with daily meals.

## 4. Amla Hair Oil

Massage amla-infused coconut oil into scalp weekly.
Prevents greying, strengthens hair, and calms the nervous system.

## SPIRITUAL PRACTICES

- Keep dried amla near your bed to absorb negative energies
- Offer amla to Goddess Durga during Navratri as a symbol of inner renewal

- Meditate on the seed of amla, visualizing a golden orb of healing light
- Mantra while consuming Amla: "May this fruit return me to the wholeness I was born with—timeless, joyful, and radiant."

## AFFIRMATION

"My light never fades. Like Amla, I hold within me the nectar of eternal renewal."

## WHY AMLA IS TRULY THE FRUIT OF IMMORTALITY

☑ Grows in dry, wild places with almost no effort

☑ Accessible year-round: fresh, dried, powdered, pickled

☑ One of the most revered Rasayanas in Ayurveda for total body rejuvenation

☑ Heals not only the body—but uplifts the ojas, the essence of life-force

# ONE-DAY HEALING MEAL PLAN WITH 11 SUPER PLANTS

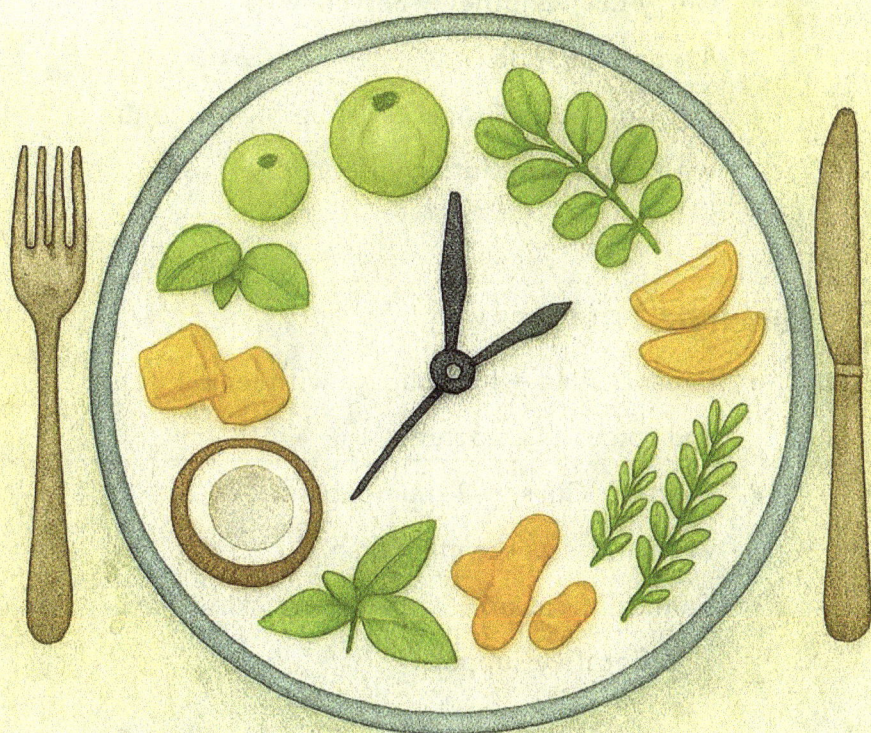

## Morning Rituals (6–8 AM)

- Neem → Brush with neem stick or rinse with neem water.
- Tulsi → Chew 3–5 fresh leaves or sip tulsi-ginger herbal tea.
- Coconut → Drink fresh coconut water for hydration and electrolytes.

## Breakfast (8–9 AM)

- Moringa Dosa/Paratha → Add moringa leaves or powder to batter/dough.
- Curry Leaf Chutney → Served with dosa/upma/poha.
- Dry Coconut + Ginger → Add grated coconut with ginger to chutney or porridge.

## Lunch (12–1 PM)

- Papaya Salad → Raw papaya with lemon, salt, and spices as a starter.
- Jackfruit Curry → Tender jackfruit cooked with spices as the main dish.
- Tamarind Rasam / Sambar → For tangy flavor and digestive support.

**Evening Snack (4–5 PM)**

- Amla Drink → Fresh juice, amla shot with honey, or dried amla candy.
- Banana → Ripe banana with a sprinkle of cinnamon for quick energy.
- Betel Leaf Digestive → Chew a fresh betel leaf with fennel seeds for breath and digestion.

**Night Ritual (9–10 PM)**

- Turmeric Golden Milk → Warm milk with turmeric and black pepper.
- Neem Mouth Rinse → Optional second use for oral care before sleep.

This structure makes each plant part of
a natural daily rhythm

CLEANSE

NOURISH

DIGEST

RESTORE

HEAL

## ABOUT THE AUTHOR

Rev. Dr. Gauri M Relan is an accomplished Holistic Healer, specializing in Natural, Vedic, and Metaphysical healing and has been healing since 1995 based on ancient Vedic philosophy of healing at Physical, Emotional, Mental and Spiritual level, so that there is total rejuvenation of physical health, emotional happiness with positive set of minds for one to finally grow spiritually. Dr. Gauri learnt various forms of Meditation and Energy healing techniques from Great Grand Masters of Reiki and Melchizedek and is a certified REIKI Master in Dr. Usui Mikao system.

Dr. Gauri did her Masters M.Sc (Botany), M.Phil (Wood Sciences & Forestry) from Himachal University Shimla, INDIA, 1992 and Ph.D from UMS, California, USA, plus numerous certification in Complimentary, Alternative & Integrative medicine from Harvard Medical School, Stanford and NIH- NCCAM (National Institutes of health - National Center for Complementary and Alternative Medicine) USA Gov. Dr Gauri was ordained as REVEREND by Wisdom of The Heart Church,

California, USA, in the year 2010. She is a certified Yoga Instructor from SVYASA University, Bangalore, a certified NLP Master Practitioner & Numerologist from American university of NLP and Certified Hypnotist from American Alliance of Hypnotists.

Dr. Gauri has authored many e-books on Apple iBooks and Amazon Kindle, APPS and many courses on UDEMY on Metaphysical self-help techniques. She has conducted numerous workshops in many corporate, many welfare clubs & societies, various schools and colleges in Bangalore. She conducts classes on YOGA, Reiki, Tarot and various Vedic and metaphysical methodologies.

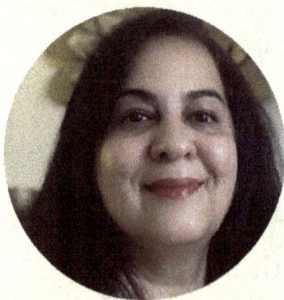

## ABOUT THE DESIGNER

Sanyukta Shanbhag is a creative designer who enjoys transforming ideas into visual experiences. She blends layout, color, and modern design tools to help stories connect with readers in meaningful ways.

# DISCLAIMER

The contents of this book are for informational purposes only and do not render any medical or psychological advice, opinion, diagnosis, or treatment. The information provided should not be used for diagnosing or treating a health problem or disease and no attempt is being made to provide diagnosis, care, treatment, or rehabilitation of individuals, or apply medical, mental health or human development principles to provide diagnosing, treating, operating, or prescribing for any human disease, pain, injury, deformity, or physical condition.

The statements and the products have not been evaluated by FDA and the services and products are not intended to diagnose, treat, cure or prevent any disease or medical condition. The information contained herein is not intended to replace a one-on-one relationship with a doctor or qualified health professional. Any techniques address only the underlying spiritual issues to address energetic blockages that may have an impact on wellness and energetic balance, facilitating the body's natural ability to bring itself to homeostasis, which may have an impact on health and well-being. This book is not a substitute for professional health care. If you have or suspect you may have a medical or psychological problem, you should consult your appropriate health care provider. Never disregard professional medical advice or delay in seeking it because of something you have read on this website. Links on this website are provided only as an informational resource, and it should not be implied that we recommend, endorse or approve of any of the content at the linked sites, nor are we responsible for their availability, accuracy or content. Any review or other matter that could be regarded as a testimonial or endorsement does not constitute a guarantee, warranty, or prediction regarding the outcome of any consultation. The testimonials on this website represent the anecdotal experience of individual consumers. Individual experiences are not a substitute for scientific research.

# MY NOTES

# MY NOTES

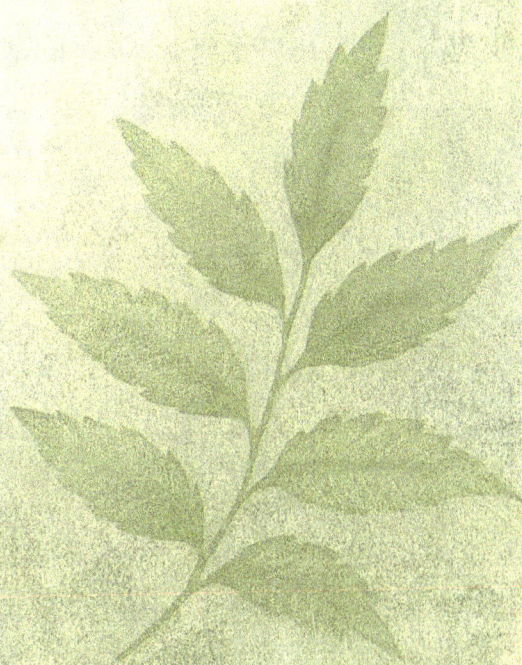

## SACRED NOURISHMENT – 11 INDIAN SUPERFOODS FOR BODY, MIND & SPIRIT

ISBN 9781734211559

Author: www.wellbeen.com

First Edition – 2025

www.ingramcontent.com/pod-product-compliance
Lightning Source LLC
Chambersburg PA
CBHW060515280326
41933CB00014B/2974